COLOR ME
PREGNANT

Quarto.com • WalterFoster.com

© 2025 Quarto Publishing Group USA Inc.
Illustrations © 2025 Veronica Carratello

Written by Rachel Hastings

First Published in 2025 by Walter Foster Publishing,
an imprint of The Quarto Group,
100 Cummings Center, Suite 265-D, Beverly, MA 01915, USA.
T (978) 282-9590 F (978) 283-2742

The information in this book is not intended to replace the medical advice of a qualified physician. Consult with your doctor before using the information in this or any health-related publication.

Walter Foster Publishing titles are also available at discount for retail, wholesale, promotional, and bulk purchase. For details, contact the Special Sales Manager by email at specialsales@quarto.com or by mail at The Quarto Group, Attn: Special Sales Manager, 100 Cummings Center, Suite 265-D, Beverly, MA 01915, USA.

29 28 27 26 25   1 2 3 4 5

ISBN: 978-0-7603-9224-9

Design and Page Layout: Mattie Wells Design LLC

Printed in China

COLOR ME PREGNANT

A Funny Activity Book for Pregnant People

Rachel Hastings

Illustrated by Veronica Carratello

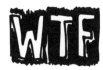

HELLO & Congratulations!

If you're reading this, it most likely means you've taken a big step toward becoming a parent:

GETTING PREGNANT.

INTRODUCTION

This is an exciting time, and also kind of scary, tiring, a little nauseating, and sometimes gassy. But we're here to help with all of that. Moral support—wise, at least.

A little bit about me: I'm Rachel, a writer and new mom in the Los Angeles area. I had my son last year and am lucky to have some close girlfriends who had kids before I did. They were so willing to share their pregnancy and parenting experiences with me, and I learned so much that I never knew before, including that "TMI" does not exist once you're pregnant or you've had a baby. Have I texted my best friend a picture of my son's poop? Yes, I have. And you'll probably get there as well. Not with me, but with your own friends. (Or with me, honestly. I'm around.)

But until then, we hope you enjoy this book. It's filled with some of the tips my friends have shared with me, some I figured out for myself, and also a bunch from more reputable sources, like doctors and stuff. There are also coloring pages, games, and puzzles to keep you occupied for the next forty weeks. I mean, it's not like you've got anything else going on, right?

Feel free to pick it up when you need a laugh, or a cry, or you're in the waiting room at your doctor's office for the hundredth time, or you wake up in the middle of the night with the inexplicable urge to do a maze. We're so excited for you and happy to be a small part of your big journey.

Also, a quick disclaimer: While sourced for accuracy, the information in this book should never come before the guidance of your medical team. Please always consult with your OB, midwife, doula, or other experts to make choices that are right for you and your pregnancy.

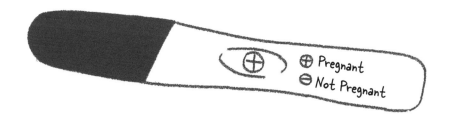

YOU & YOUR PREGNANCY

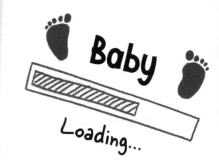

Baby

Loading...

Since this book is all about you and your pregnancy—the good, the bad, and the nauseous—tell us all about it!

Hi, my name is _____ !

I am currently _____ weeks pregnant.

My due date is _____ .

Physically, I am feeling _____ .

Emotionally, I am feeling _____ .

The best thing about pregnancy so far has been

_____ .

The worst thing about pregnancy so far has been

_____ .

Thinking about becoming a parent makes me

_____ .

My baby is going to be as cute as a _____ , if not cuter.

DROPPING THE BABY BOMBSHELL

Okay, so maybe this isn't *exactly* how you broke the news, or maybe it is! If you've got a buddy nearby, hand this page to them so they can write your answers in. Or if you're flying solo, do your best to fill them in without peeking at the story first.

I was out to brunch with _____ when I decided it was
(NAME OF A FRIEND)

finally time to break the news. Once our _____
(DRINK, PLURAL)

came, I told them, "I'm pregnant!" They were so excited that they spit the whole

_____ out. They then bumped into a waiter who was
(SAME DRINK, BUT SINGULAR)

carrying a full tray of _____ , and it went everywhere.
(FOOD, PLURAL)

All of a sudden, a _____ , _____ ,
(TYPE OF DOG)   (ANOTHER TYPE OF DOG)

and _____ came out of nowhere and ate all of it!
(ANOTHER TYPE OF DOG)

The manager was furious, but after we explained what happened, they gave us two

_____ on the house. Weirdest part is, this has happened
(BRUNCH DISH, PLURAL)

_____ times now!
(NUMBER HIGHER THAN ONE)

NAUSEA NAUSEA NAUSEA

See how many words you can create using the phrase

"I feel unbelievably nauseous."

Like, "fun" or "sauna." And I hope it goes without saying that we don't think being nauseous in a sauna would be fun.

GET THAT SALAD AWAY FROM ME!

If some of your favorite foods are grossing you out right now, don't worry. You will love broccoli again, we just know it. But for now, unscramble these common pregnancy food aversions.

GESG _____

AETM _____

NONSOI _____

YPSCI ODOFS _____

HIFS _____

RAYID RUTPDOSC _____

ILACRG _____

OFECEF _____

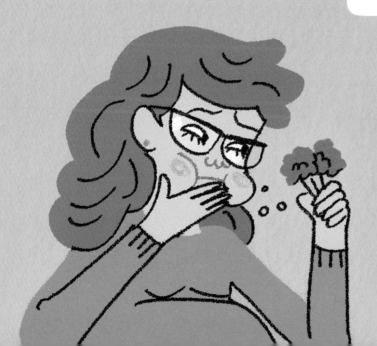

Answers on page 91.

IT'S 12 A.M., DO YOU KNOW WHERE YOUR CURLY FRIES ARE?

It's midnight, and you're craving curly fries from the place all the way across town. Will they be worth it? *Yes.* But is it a real trek for your partner or friend or delivery driver? *Also yes.*

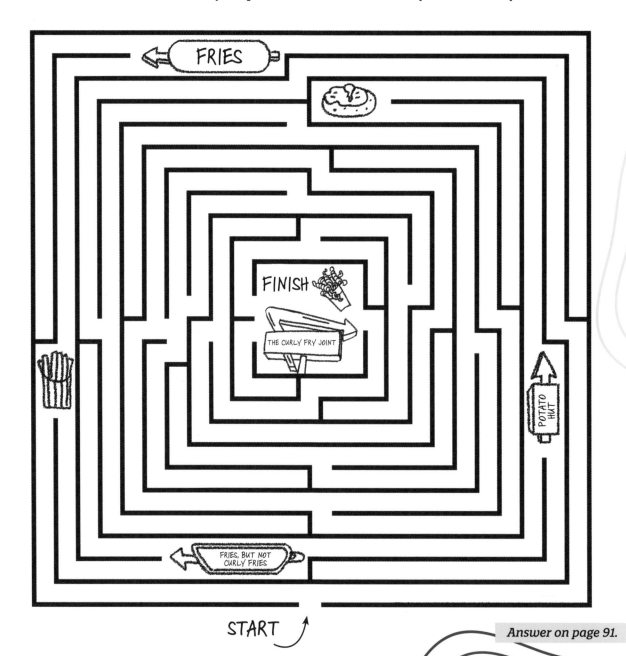

FRIES

FINISH

THE CURLY FRY JOINT

POTATO HUT

FRIES, BUT NOT CURLY FRIES

START

Answer on page 91.

PEE ON THIS STICK

Now that you've gotten the news, calm your anxious mind by coloring this in.

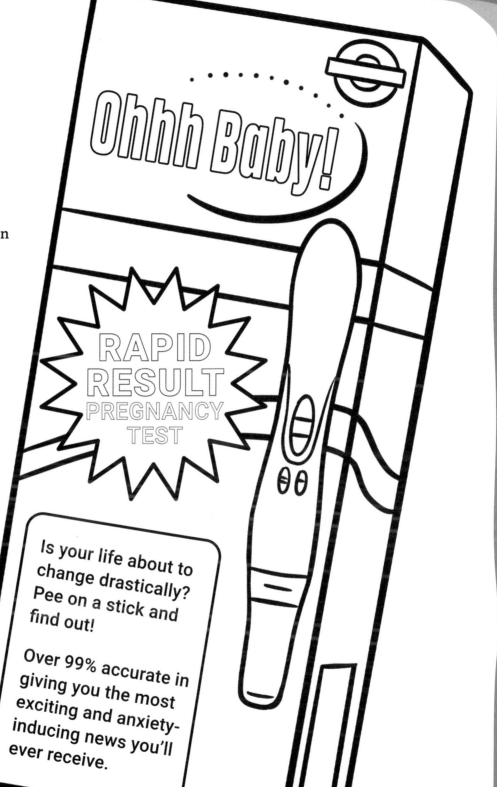

TRUE OR FALSE: WHAT'S OFF-LIMITS

You may have heard that you'll have to quit your morning cup of coffee once you get pregnant. But do you really? Test your knowledge to find out! Circle true or false below. But, as always, check with your health care practitioner!

1. Caffeine is completely off-limits during pregnancy.

   True   False

2. Same goes for alcohol.

   True   False

3. How about sushi? No-go, right?

   True   False

4. Tobacco is definitely a no?

   True   False

5. Marijuana has got to be a no, amiright?

   True   False

6. I can have soft cheeses, right? I love a good brie.

   True   False

7. I am and/or live with a grill master and can definitely chow down on a rare steak.

   True   False

8. At least my trusty deli meat sandwiches are fine for all those rushed lunches.

   True   False

Answers on page 91.

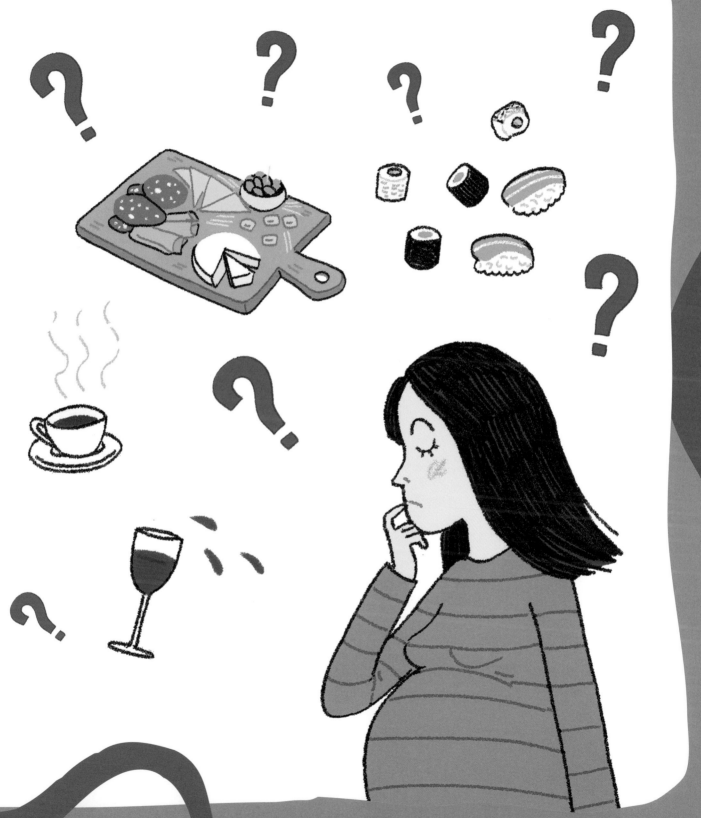

WHAT ALL THE PREGNANCY TEST SYMBOLS MEAN

If you're reading this, it's likely you've already successfully taken, and read, a pregnancy test. But just in case you need a refresher, here's what the symbols mean. Color these in!

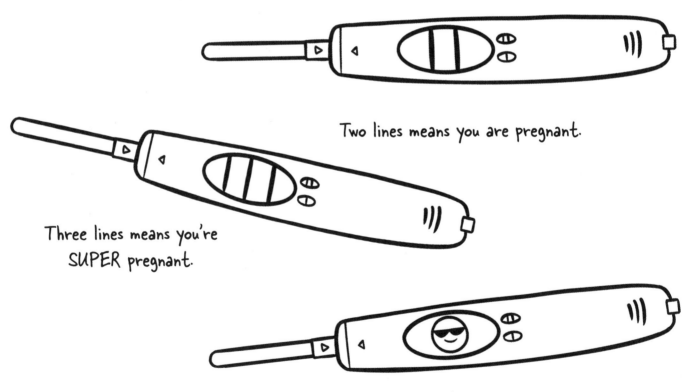

One line means you're not pregnant.

Two lines means you are pregnant.

Three lines means you're
SUPER pregnant.

Sunglasses means you're pregnant
with a chill baby.

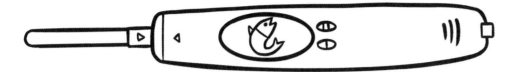

Fish means your baby will be an
Olympic swimmer.

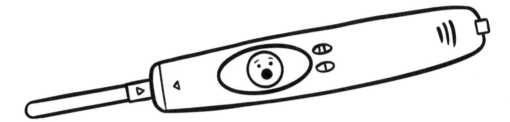

Shocked face means you're
pregnant with twins.

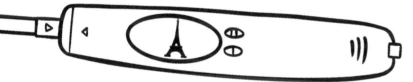

Eiffel Tower means your baby will
become a pastry chef (in which
case, please call us).

The Prince symbol means your baby
will either become a rock icon or
look great in purple.

SO MANY BOOKS

There are so many books for pregnant people. But some of them are for partners too! Can you spot the dfferences between the two books?

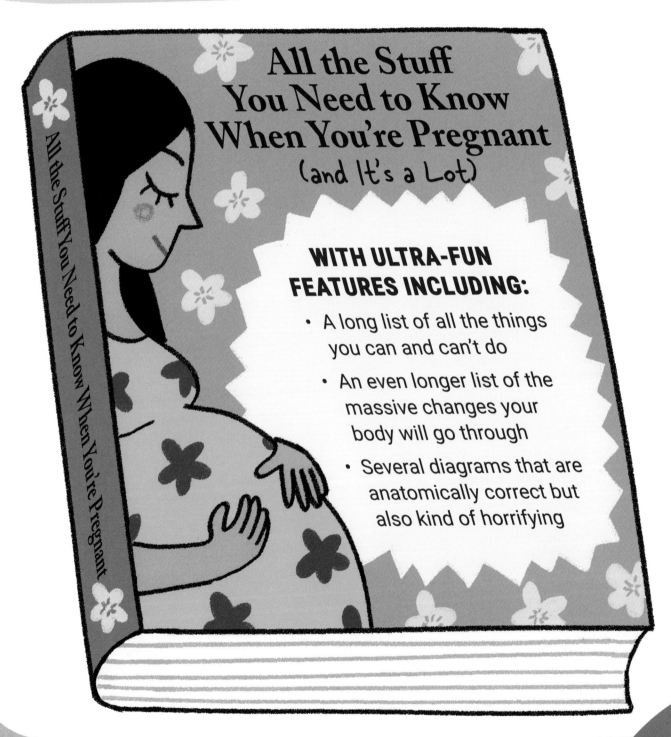

All the Stuff You Need to Know When You're Pregnant (and It's a Lot)

WITH ULTRA-FUN FEATURES INCLUDING:

- A long list of all the things you can and can't do
- An even longer list of the massive changes your body will go through
- Several diagrams that are anatomically correct but also kind of horrifying

All the Stuff You Need to Know When You're Pregnant

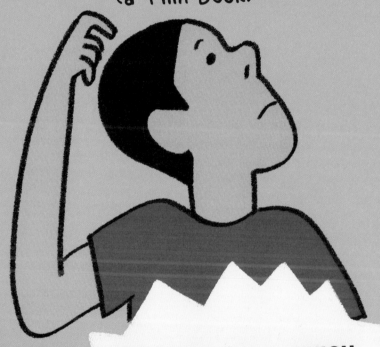

All the Stuff You Need to Know When Your Partner Is Pregnant

(a Thin Book)

WITH ONE TOPIC, WHICH IS PRETTY MUCH JUST:

- How to ask your partner what they need for 40 weeks and then do all of those things

ALL THE FEELS

Finding out you're pregnant can make you feel so many things. Here is a non-exhaustive list of them! Circle the words in the puzzle on the next page; and hey, we're here for you.

HAPPY	DELIGHTED	TERRIFIED
EXCITED	EMPOWERED	ECSTATIC
NERVOUS	SHOCKED	PANICKED
SCARED	APPREHENSIVE	ELATED
OVERWHELMED	OVERJOYED	SURPRISED
ANXIOUS	THRILLED	LUCKY
GIDDY	FORTUNATE	

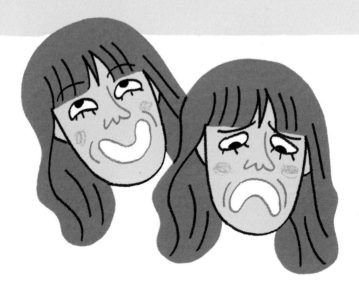

```
P I H F B I T U Q A E R Y W R N M Q C W X B D
B A V O Y E C S T A T I C J R N G X M T B E N
F H N K U Y F R W K E Y S Y S E U R D V T L N
N G C I H J Y U H X U S H O C K E D R A D I V
N U J L C O S O O U G T J N T G M L L Y H U L
L Q H S B K W R Q D G R K H I F N E A J N E A
D T F F N D E A S U R P R I S E D H I D K A P
O I H A Y Y F D U R B M T A C K K Q H K P C P
X K L T L E Y V N F S M S M O W K X B Y F H R
P V X P K D S H K N X U P T Z U A V K H F D E
M O J K D H X T J G O D E L I G H T E D U W H
T M Q I Q T A Y N V X E L F J E V P V U W C E
U D G A M H A P R D H M C S K O Y D N L Q N N
K E F G C R H E P V O P E R T V W I U H N Y S
C C W T L I N S Y Y A O Y W D E R P O N B U I
T P Y I M L D C D I Z W Q L Z R B V F T O Y V
U T N M O L L A B V N E A E R J J W I I V V E
X A B K W E V R U N Z R J X W O C Y X E Z Y I
W Q Z U H D I E O J S E N C P Y C N S S J R I
H V Q R L O W D M Q X D O I P E A M O K S S S
F O V E R W H E L M E D I T I D E I T G W O K
F O R T U N A T E K C F B E J J R I U Y Q Y L
K F V D O T E R R I F I E D A Y A Y U T F E G
```

Answers on page 92.

IF YOU COULD BE ANYWHERE

Sometimes you just need a mental escape. If you could be anywhere right now, where would you be? Take a moment and draw what you might see out of your window. A beach, a pizza, a pizza on a beach.

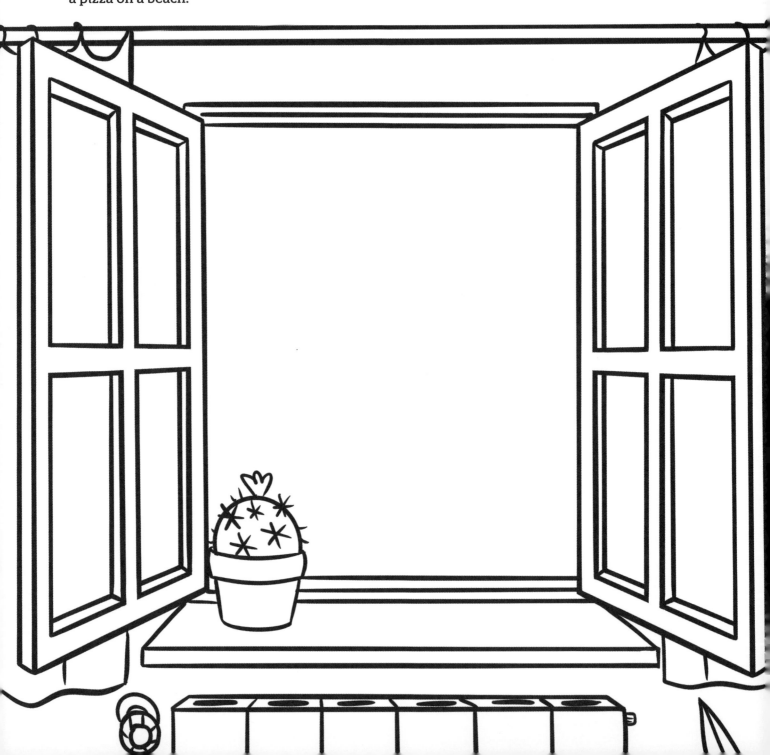

FIND YOUR PHONE

Pregnancy brain is real, and it's not your fault. You know you had your phone at some point. But where did you put it? Your underwear drawer? Out with the mail? Make your way through the maze to find out where it is this time.

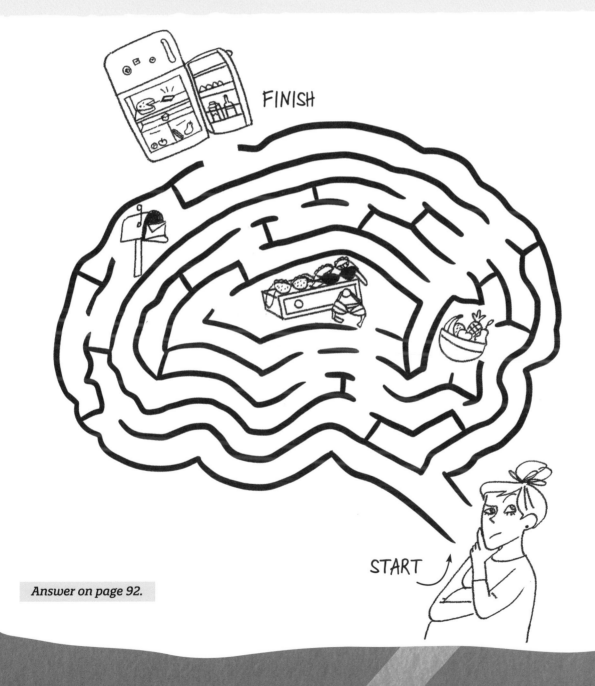

FINISH

START

Answer on page 92.

VISITING YOUR O.B.F.F.

You and your OB, midwife, or other care provider are going to be spending *a lot* of quality time together. Make your (many) visits easier with the following tips, and color them in, if you like.

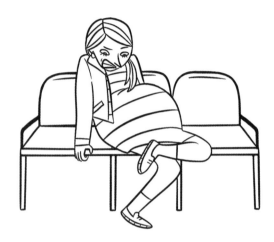

Get familiar with their office, because you're gonna be there a lot! While you'll be visiting your provider once a month early on, by the time you hit thirty-six weeks, you'll be there once a week.

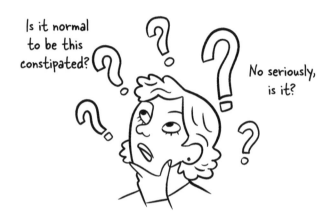

Is it normal to be this constipated?

No seriously, is it?

Write down questions for your next appointment as they come to you so you don't forget them. (Bonus tip: Your phone's Notes app is great for this!)

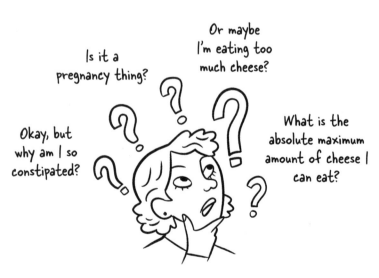

Or maybe I'm eating too much cheese?

Is it a pregnancy thing?

Okay, but why am I so constipated?

What is the absolute maximum amount of cheese I can eat?

Don't be afraid to ask too many questions, either—your provider is there to support you!

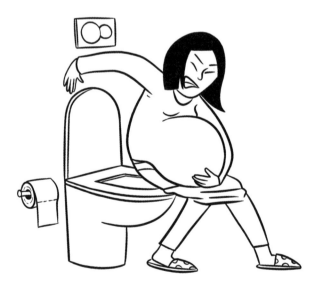

You'll probably have to give a urine sample at each visit, so make sure to space out your pre-appointment bathroom trips.

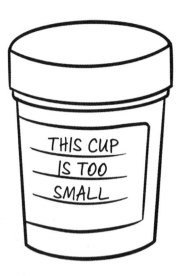

Also, the more pregnant you get, the harder it is to pee in the cup. (Sorry.)

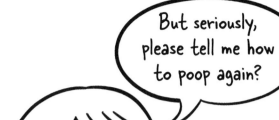

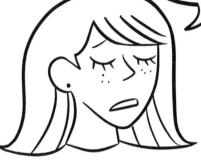

Advocate for yourself. If you feel like something's off, make sure your provider hears you.

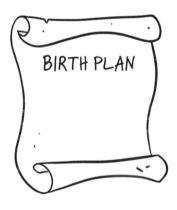

Talk birth plan. As your due date nears, make sure you and your provider are on the same page about your preferences.

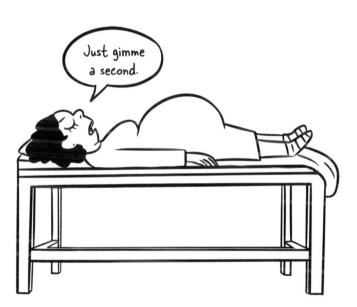

When they tell you to sit up at the end of the appointment, it's okay if it takes kind of a long time. (This is mostly a third-trimester tip!)

ACTUALLY, REALLY GREAT THINGS ABOUT BEING PREGNANT

It's good to remember pregnancy is not all nausea, heartburn, and memory loss! Unscramble these words to find out what pregnancy perks you have to look forward to!

ON REDOPI _____ _____

RATEG AIRH _____ _____

GNOTSR SNLIA _____ _____

TSRNGRESA RAE ECIN _____ _____ _____ _____

BBAY KKSIC _____ _____

TASILCE BSTIAWDANS _____ _____

GNIFELE REWPODEEM _____ _____

OS NAYM PNAS ___ _____ _____

Answers on page 92.

24

WOW, SO PEOPLE JUST TALK TO YOU WHEN YOU'RE PREGNANT!?

I mean, getting advice from random people at the grocery store might as well be an official pregnancy symptom. But maybe some of it's good? Hopefully? Either way, we wanna hear about it.

The best piece of advice I've gotten is _____.

The worst piece of advice I've gotten is _____.

The nicest thing a stranger has said to me is _____.

The weirdest thing a stranger has said to me is _____.

The nicest compliment I've gotten is _____.

The strangest comment I've gotten is _____.

Current count of people who have tried to touch my stomach:

_____.

When people try to touch my stomach, I would like to

_____.

HOW BIG THE BABY FEELS, WEEK BY WEEK

We all have an app that tells us how big the baby is each week. But how big does the baby *feel*? Feel free to color in your metaphorical baby week by week.

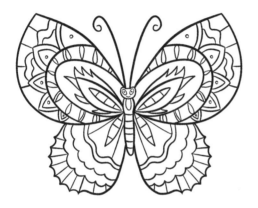

Weeks 0–12: A sweet lil' butterfly

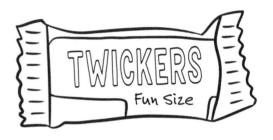

Weeks 13–20: A fun-size candy bar

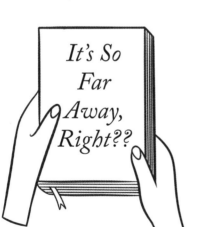

Weeks 20–24: A parenting book you'll get around to reading at some point

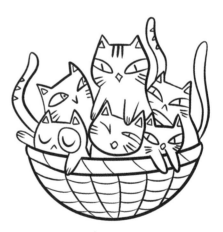

Weeks 25–28: A basket of very active kittens

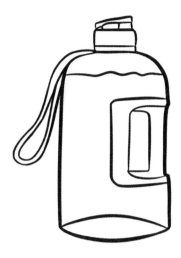

Weeks 29–32: The giant jug of water you're supposed to drink every day

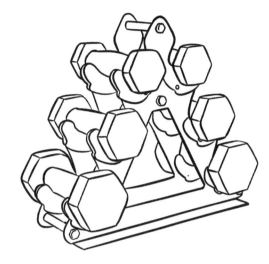

Weeks 33–36: A small rack of dumbbells

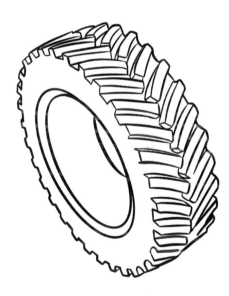

Weeks 37–38: One of those big tires that they use in weightlifting competitions

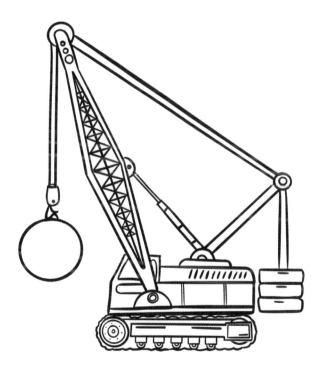

Weeks 39–40: An actual wrecking ball

YOUR PREGNANCY SCRAPBOOK

Here are a couple of pages you can fill with all your pregnancy milestones.
You can draw them, or print out photos and tape them in, or hey, you can go
full Martha Stewart and make a whole craft project out of it.

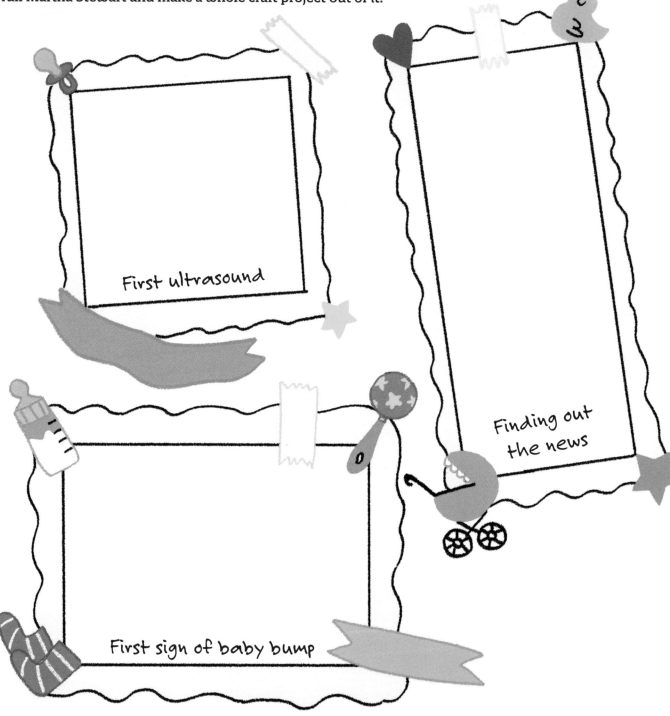

First ultrasound

Finding out
the news

First sign of baby bump

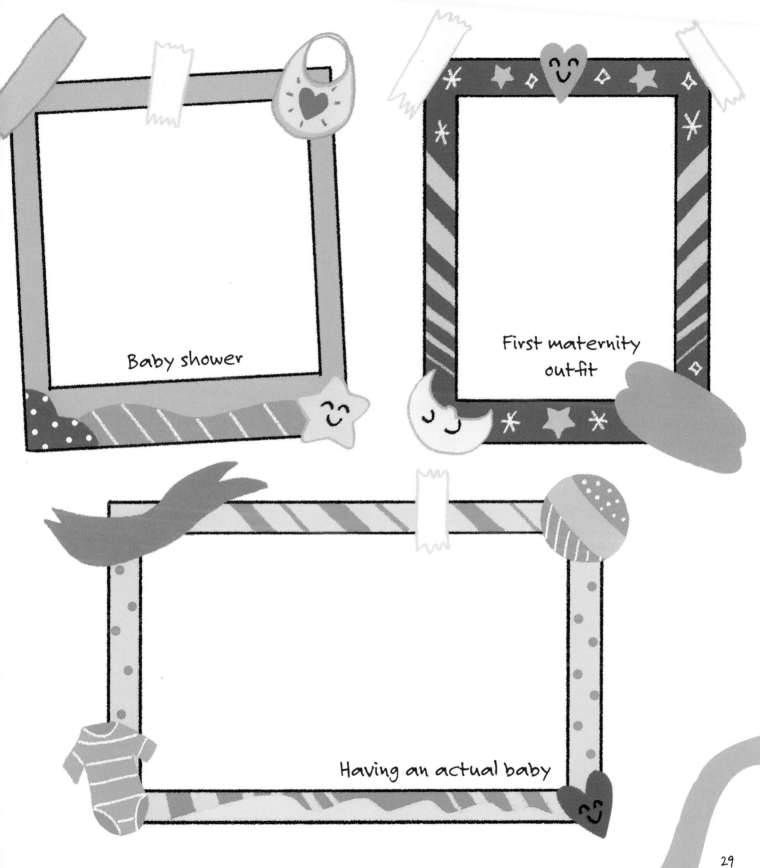

Baby shower

First maternity outfit

Having an actual baby

29

WAIT, I CAN'T GO SKYDIVING?

We know it's hard to give up some of your favorite activities while you're pregnant. But we promise you'll be able to do each and every one of these things again at some point. Your trapeze lessons aren't going anywhere.

WATERSKIING

SKYDIVING

RACE CAR DRIVING

BMX BIKING

GYMNASTICS

SCUBA DIVING

RIDING ROLLER
COASTERS

TRAPEZE

TRAMPOLINING

RUGBY

TIGHTROPE WALKING

AXE THROWING

ARCHERY

FENCING

WRESTLING

CLIFF DIVING

POLE VAULTING

PARKOUR

SNOWBOARDING

SLEEPING ON YOUR
STOMACH

```
H R E V V A G T P Z R W S F S D V F S S U P J
F A O L Q P O H A V W V O F E L T E D S S K T
R S N O W B O A R D I N G Z Y Y H N P S D P R
A A G Y M N A S T I C S E E Q T G C Q O R O F
H H C N T P B A F P V P E H S T B I D G F L P
A X C E P R T F O J A Q U M Q W M N L K G E A
H T J N C T A U U R X P H L T B C G O N B V R
L I V A H A Q M T Q E K S C B X M W I M K A K
W T I G H T R O P E W A L K I N G V K P J U O
A U M C Z Z U D T O E F R W Y K I P Z Z F L U
T T L O J V Q A R D L W N S R D F D R I Z T R
E C M S B V O Z C I H I M H F E I I D X T I E
R U Y A C G Q H Y Q V Q N F L I S V K X N N Y
S W D Y A Q P B Q O J I I I T J Q T I X X G N
K K I L F G G A K F O L N E N R X I L N N I Y
I S A N H U P I K H C M P G D G H N E I G K A
I Q A T R V E S E O K V K E Q U M P Z A N J R
N S C U B A D I V I N G P A G H F J G P K G C
G R I D I N G R O L L E R C O A S T E R S K H
E B M B M X B I K I N G C J E L M O Y A I P E
K I P A X E T H R O W I N G I G M J O S S A R
S L E E P I N G O N Y O U R S T O M A C H G Y
W G S P C M X A D C P V J Y L S D L M I L U U
```

Answers on page 92.

WHERE SHOULD YOU 'MOON?

Planning a trip before baby arrives but not quite sure where to take that cute little (or big) bump? We can help! Take this quiz and then turn to page 93 to find out where we think you should babymoon!

1. **What is your current energy level?**
   a. Miraculously energetic!
   b. Eh, I can get around
   c. Girl, I'm tired
   d. Zzzzzzzzzzzz

2. **The thought of going on a plane makes you feel:**
   a. Fine!
   b. Okay, sure
   c. I mean, not great
   d. 1,000% no

3. **Which nap location sounds the most relaxing?**
   a. Hammock in the woods
   b. Museum bench
   c. Lounge chair
   d. Any horizontal surface

4. **Which of the following outfits sounds the most comfortable?**
   a. Windbreaker and bike shorts
   b. Shirtdress
   c. Bathing suit
   d. "Comfortable" lol

5. **How much walking are you up for?**
   a. All the walking!
   b. I can manage a bit
   c. Minimal
   d. "Walking" lol

6. **Proximity to a good restaurant is:**
   a. Not essential
   b. Incredibly essential
   c. Helpful, but I'm not picky
   d. Do they deliver?

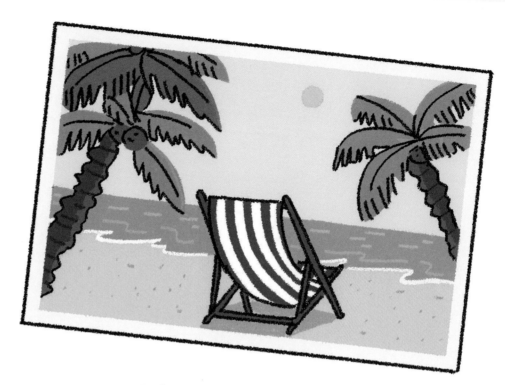

7. **What's your top babymoon priority?**
   a. Great scenery
   b. Great culture
   c. Great beaches
   d. Great pillows

8. **After this trip, you want to feel:**
   a. Invigorated
   b. Educated
   c. Relaxed
   d. Even slightly less sleepy,
      if that's possible

Answers on page 93.

LESSER-KNOWN PREGNANCY SYMPTOMS

While nausea and fatigue are common symptoms of pregnancy, there are a whole bunch of others you might not know about. And a surprising number of them are nose-related! Color this!

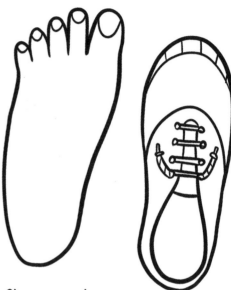

Change in shoe size

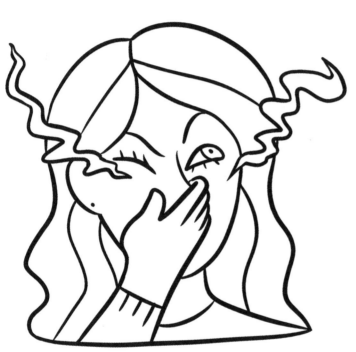

Heightened sense of smell

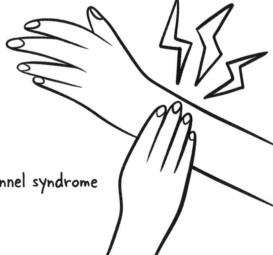

Carpal tunnel syndrome

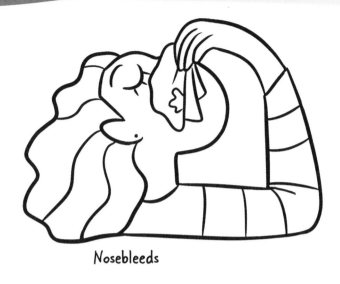

Nosebleeds

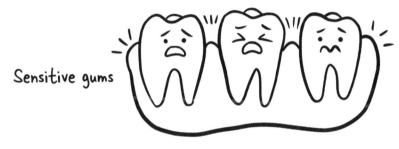

Sensitive gums

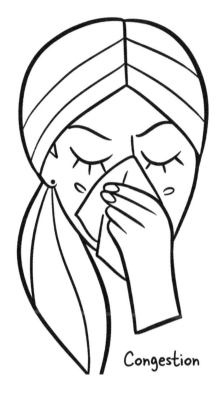

Congestion

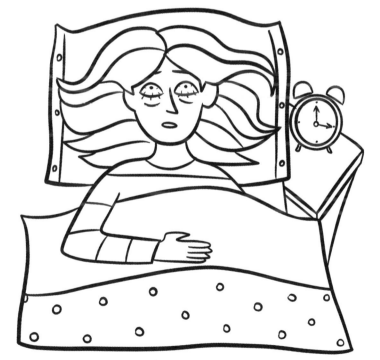

Insomnia

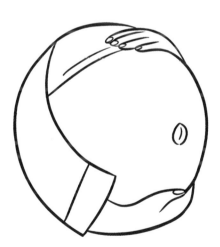

Changing belly button

THINGS THAT MAKE YOU PEE NOW, APPARENTLY

Unscramble all the things that make you pee and, while you're thinking, practice those Kegels.

EIGNZESN _____

CGHONUIG _____

UGNIHLAG _____

DGENIBN _____

NUNGIRN _____

IFTILNG _____

KAGNILW _____

YTEGRVINHE _____

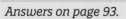

Answers on page 93.

SHOW US YOUR BUMP

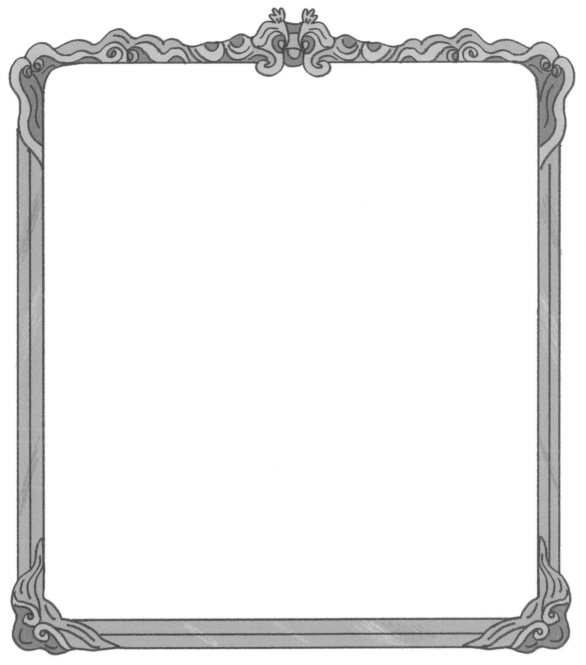

Draw your baby bump mirror selfie! (And hey, if it's just a pregnant
stick figure, that's great. You're doing great.)

YOUR MATERNITY LOOK: RIHANNA VS. REALITY

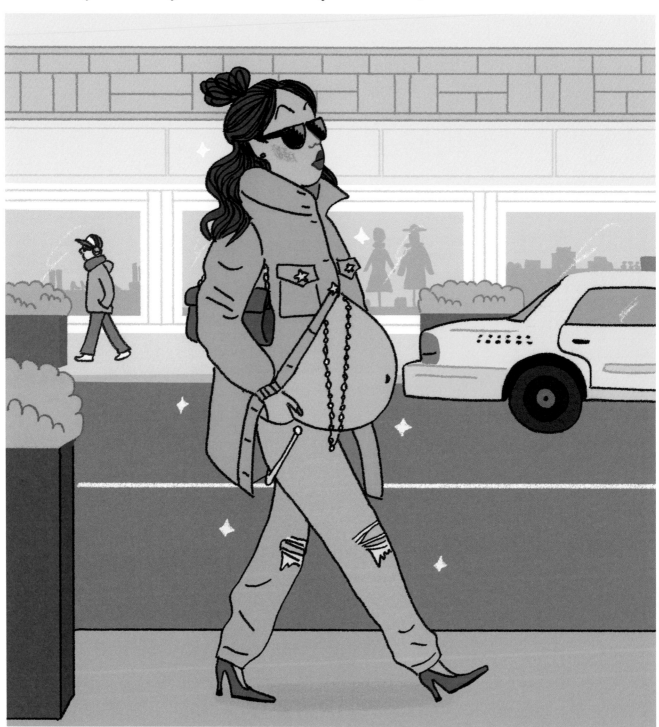

Spot the differences between what you thought your maternity look was going to be and what it really is. (And, we can't stress this enough, you're doing *great*.)

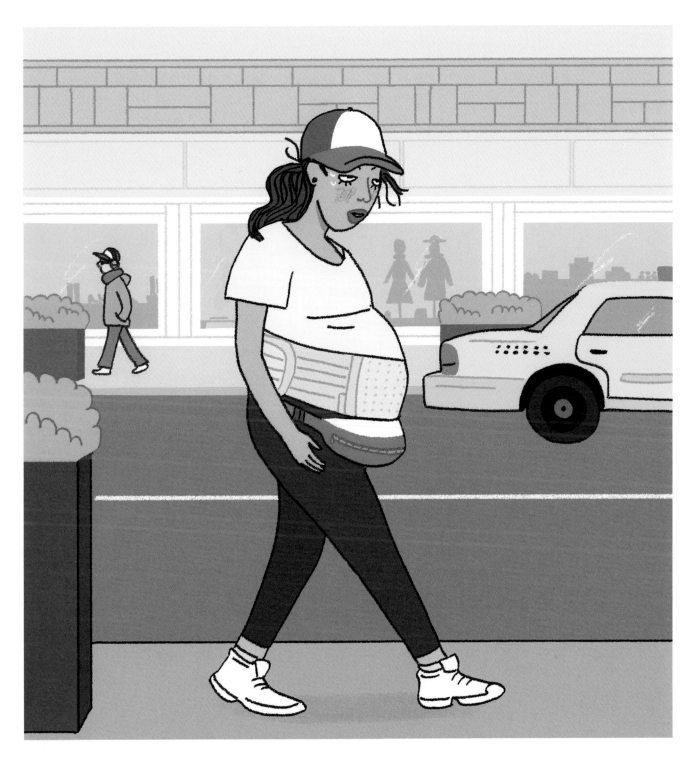

SO WHAT ARE THEY DOING IN THERE?

While it might seem like the answer is "not much," babies are literally developing from two cells into a whole person. But what's actually going on? Test your knowledge and circle true or false!

1. Babies can hear in the womb.

   True   False

2. They can also see.

   True   False

3. Babies can taste what you're eating while you're pregnant.

   True   False

4. Babies can specifically tell if you're eating chicken tikka masala.

   True   False

5. Babies sleep in the womb.

   True   False

6. They dream too.

   True   False

7. Babies can smell as early as 8 weeks.

   True   False

8. They can also hold their nose if something is stinky.

   True   False

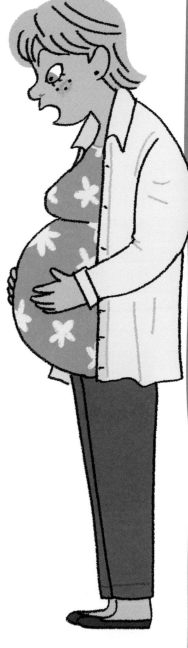

Answers on page 93.

TAKING CARE OF YOU

It turns out growing a whole human is kind of a lot of work, so be sure to take care of yourself, mama. Relax by coloring this in.

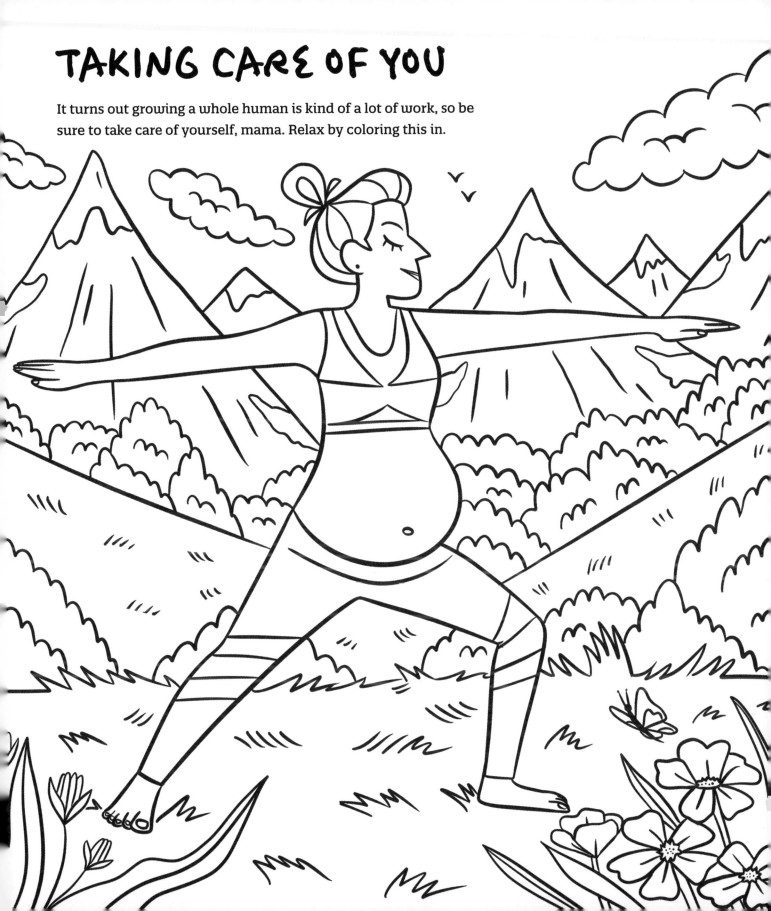

ALL THE PILLOWS

When you're pregnant, it can be hard to sleep (or even sit) comfortably. Luckily, there are truly so many pillows for that. Here are a few to try out! Did you know the next most relaxing thing after sleeping is coloring? We made that up, but color these in!

Wedge: For bump support, back support, or between your knees

Butterfly: Bump support on both sides

J-shaped: Head, belly, and knee support on one side

C-shaped: Like the J, but with added back support

U-shaped: The big one. Full support on both sides

Regular ol' body pillow: No-frills, classic comfort

Surrounded-by-puppies: Did we make this one up? Possibly! Does that make it any less cute? Absolutely not

Car jack: Okay, this one isn't real either, but it gets so hard to sit up!

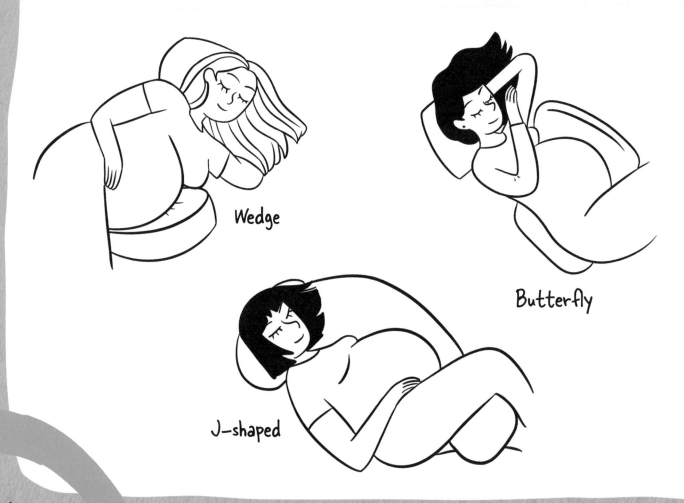

Wedge

Butterfly

J-shaped

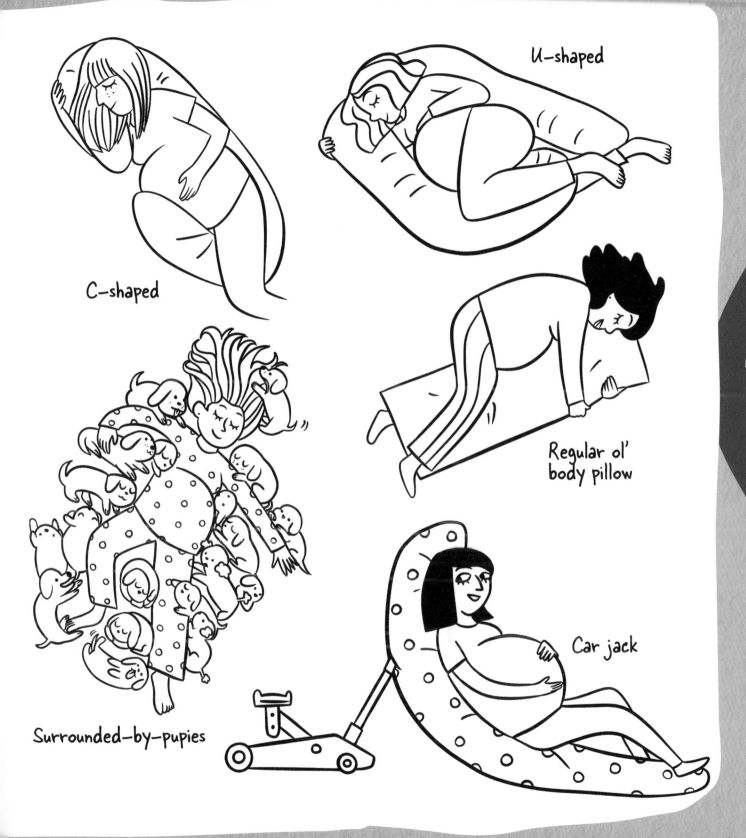

C-shaped

U-shaped

Regular ol' body pillow

Surrounded-by-pupies

Car jack

HERE'S YOUR KICKER

Once you're about halfway through your pregnancy, you'll probably be feeling those little kicks. Here's a list of things your baby is definitely not doing in there . . . or are they??

SOCCER

KARATE

KICKBOXING

CHORUS LINE

KICKBALL

TAP DANCING

CAPOEIRA

HACKY SACK

BREAKDANCING

SALSA DANCING

DISCO

STEP AEROBICS

ZUMBA

GYMNASTICS

BATON TWIRLING

DRUMMING

BADMINTON

SAYING "KEEP IT DOWN
OUT THERE"

TIDYING UP

MOSHING

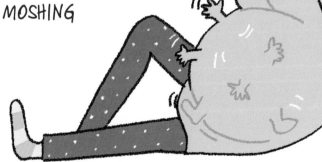

```
S A Y I N G K E E P I T D O W N O U T T H E R E W
D I I O M H T W Z M N L U R K N O V W D M A L S N
N U E T Y H A K U I Z B F Z V P Q D D J O J R G W
Y X W C W B D M V Y O A E S P L R G I D T C R E N
A E G I E U A Y M G J A M F Z V N K T E H I S P Z
Q E F J G K O T S T E P A E R O B I C S T X H R M
H O K X W W T A O C H T M L A L U Z K N O P Y T D
A C B F X I D M M N P P K N T Y M J Z U M B A L O
V F S Y L D X M Y C T A P D A N C I N G P J C S J
X U C B G S O Q J B J W M S B G C U J U S C E O X
K B G Y M N A S T I C S I S N P L L T Y R T I D N
B R E A K D A N C I N G V R B A D M I N T O N B P
O K E L I Z Q A K E D N R S L M V R R K F O O Y T
R D T D E V R Z X L M I M U P I U Q Z L C S H F P
B F T K L I T K F L S V B O P T N A N R E A L H X
O W M B E F V M I Z Z S C G S W J G U N F L F A A
T H O O Z B B C J C U W G B B H Z H I R A S D C V
U O P E R Z H Z D I K U A K F W I L V B D A P K W
V A U F I L J L F P E B Q Y O Y S N K A R D S Y N
C U I G D F K Y O B B R O J C U M C G O U A O S E
C B L V N I S A P U N G H X R W I S M Y M N C A S
Q L O G L B S F R N E X F O I K C I X V M C C C N
T E F S Q K M C X A T N H F J N L K T E I I E K Q
F K Q I W S M T O N T C R U P L G Z T Z N N R Y G
T I D Y I N G U P F T E U T R A U U Y L G G R U H
```

Answers on page 93.

MATERNITY

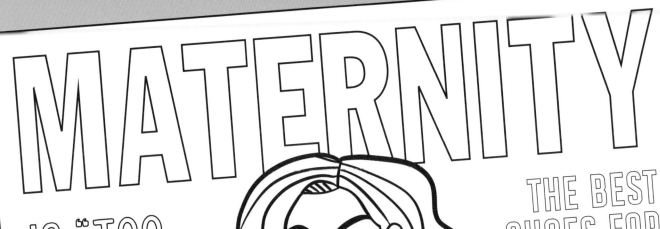

IS "TOO
HIGH–
WAISTED"
A THING?
(NO.)

THE BEST
SHOES FOR
PREGNANCY

And yes, they're
all Birkenstocks.

MATERNITY
MAGAZINE

Color this, you cover girl!

HOW TO
TAKE A
PAIR OF
SWEATPANTS
FROM DAY
TO NIGHT

by just leaving them on.

ARE YOU THERE, FEET?
IT'S ME, PREGNANT.

You haven't seen your feet in months. Draw the things you can no longer pick up and color this in!

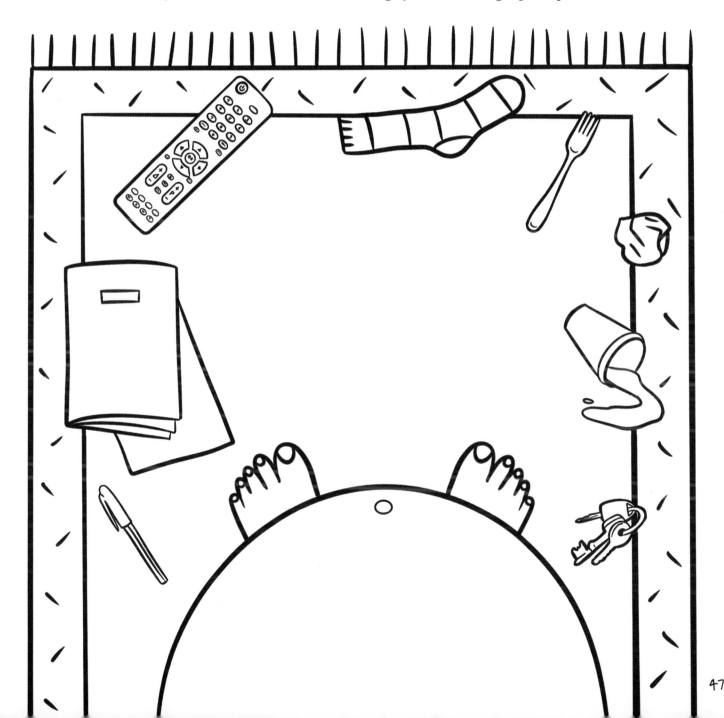

WAIT, NEW UNDIES TOO??

Sooner or later, there will come a point when your pre-pregnancy bras and panties won't get the job done. So, what's your maternity underwear vibe? Let's find out! Take the quiz and then turn to page 94.

1. **Pre-pregnancy, what was your bra of choice?**
   a. Racerback
   b. Bralette
   c. Pushup
   d. Anything that looks like it was made from a curtain

2. **How about panties?**
   a. Boy short
   b. Bikini
   c. Thong
   d. The curtain thing again, but for panties

3. **If you had to choose one color, your bras and panties would be:**
   a. Black
   b. Gray
   c. Red
   d. Off-white

4. **And fabric?**
   a. Spandex-y
   b. 100% cotton
   c. Silk, mesh, whatever looks cute!
   d. I don't care, as long as there's a lot of it

5. **The most important feature of underwear is:**
   a. Support
   b. Comfort
   c. Appearance
   d. Coverage, coverage, coverage

6. **How active are you these days?**
   a. Very
   b. Not very
   c. Extremely, but mostly in the bedroom
   d. Ha!

7. **If/when you do move, what's your activity of choice?**
   a. Running
   b. Maaaaaybe some yoga
   c. Sex, obviously
   d. None of the above

8. **What's your favorite design detail?**
   a. Sporty bands or patterns
   b. I'm not particular about design
   c. Sexy cutouts
   d. Tasteful frills. Or any kind of frills, honestly

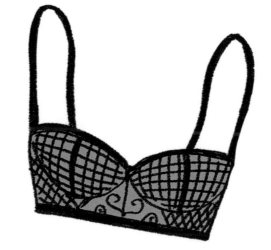

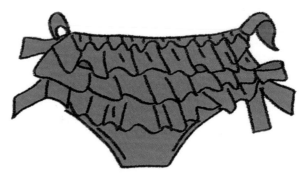

Answers on page 94.

AN ODE TO BOOBS

My boobs, they have begun to change
They're getting bigger every day
My bras, they barely can contain
Will my shirts ever look the same again?
Squishy melons, big balloons
I sure hope they stop growing soon
But in the mirror, I look twice
Because actually, they look pretty nice

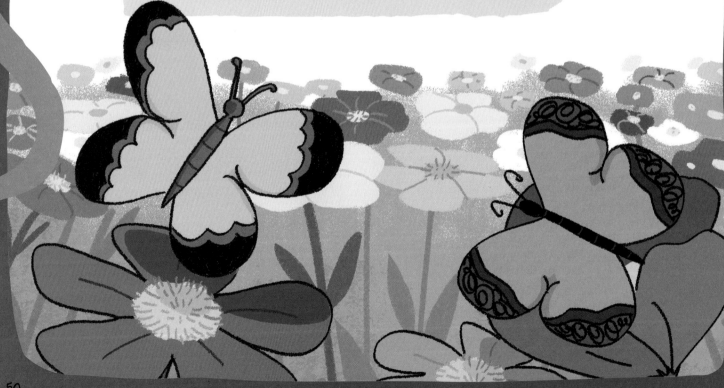

THE MOODS, THEY ARE A-CHANGIN'

It's not your fault you can feel happy and sad and angry and happy and angry and sad and sad-angry all within the span of five minutes. Make your way through this maze of emotions.

START

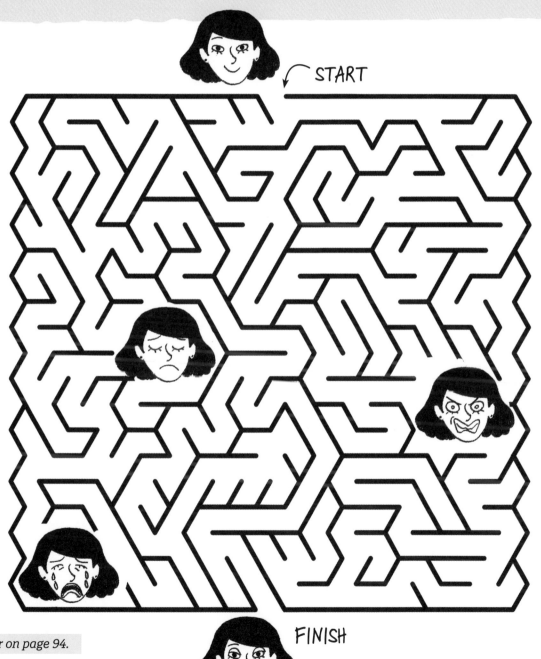

Answer on page 94.

FINISH

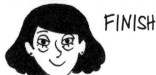

REMEMBER SLEEP?

Spot the differences between how you used to sleep and now, and then color them in!
And also, we're sorry.

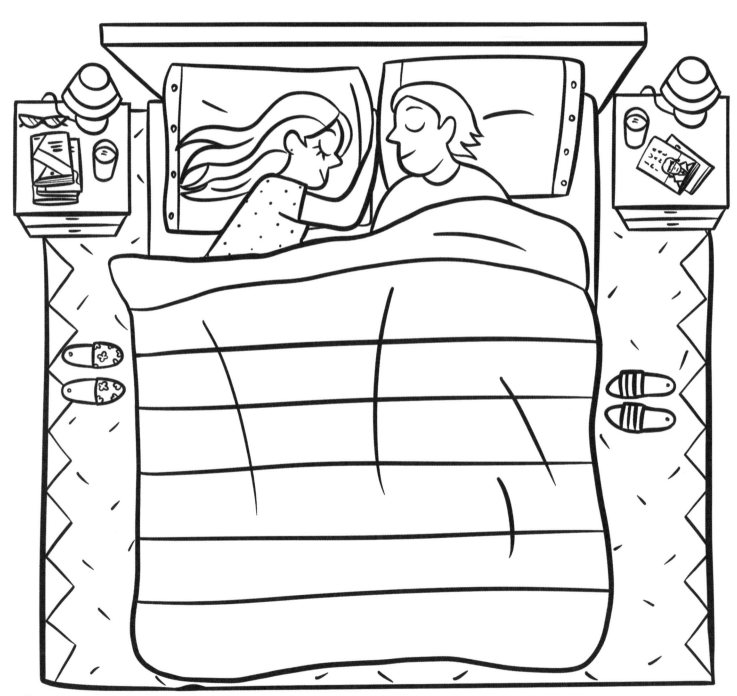

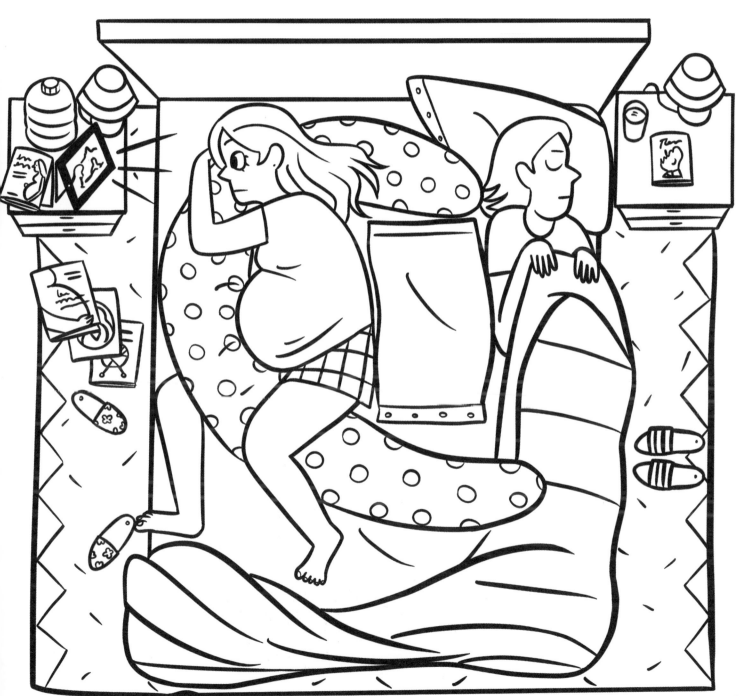

A LULLABY FOR INSOMNIA

If you're reading this in the middle of the night and have already watched more than one episode of *Shark Tank*, try singing yourself this lullaby to the tune of "Rock-a-Bye Baby."

I'm wide awake

And it's 3 a.m.

Wish I could sleep

Until 9 or 10

But it's not happ'ning

Even though I'm tired

I'll go eat some cheese

Hope it's not expired

IT'S A BABY!

Sure, you've seen an ultrasound of your little one, but draw what you think your cutie might look like when they're finally here.

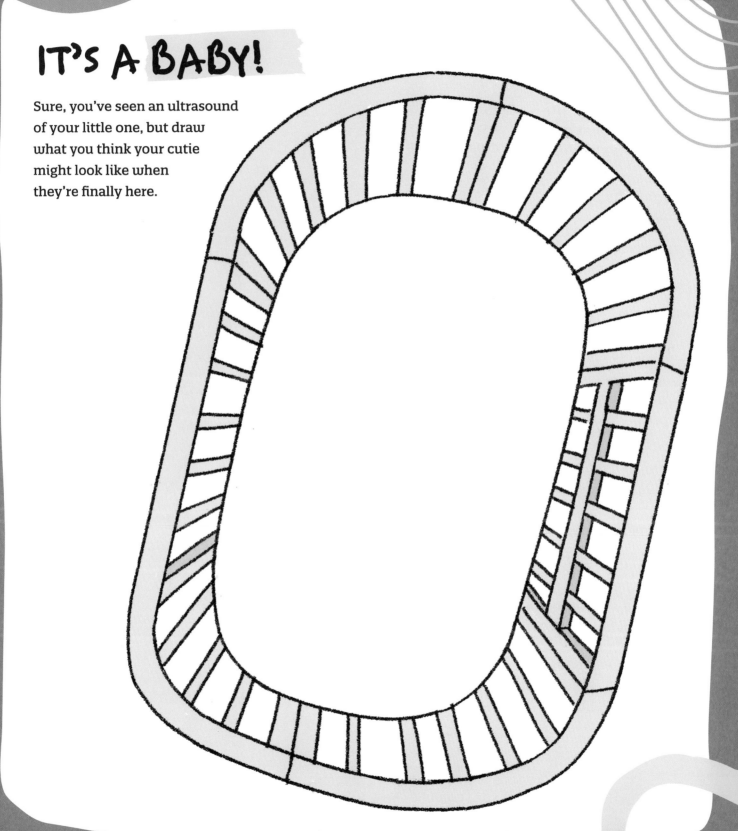

WAYS YOU CAN MOVE (IF YOU WANT TO)

If you're feeling up to it (and are cleared by your doctor), it can be great to stay moving in ways that are still comfortable for you and your bump. And we don't care what anyone says, those belly support bands look *very* cool. But if you're not feeling motivated right now, that's OK! Color these in, instead.

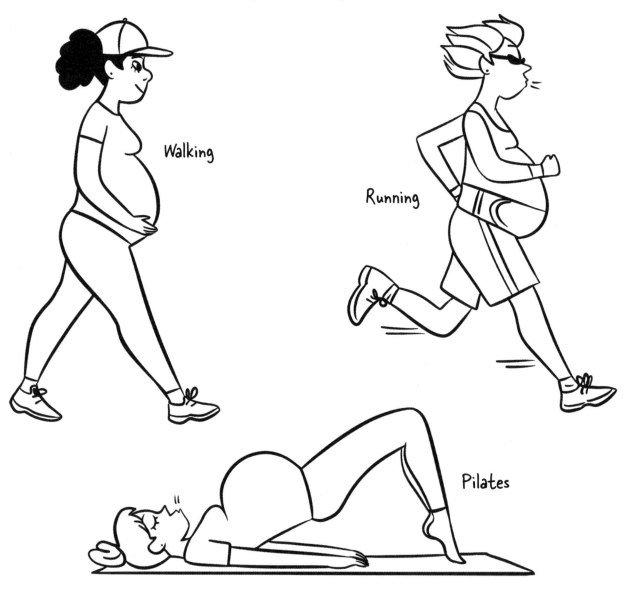

Walking

Running

Pilates

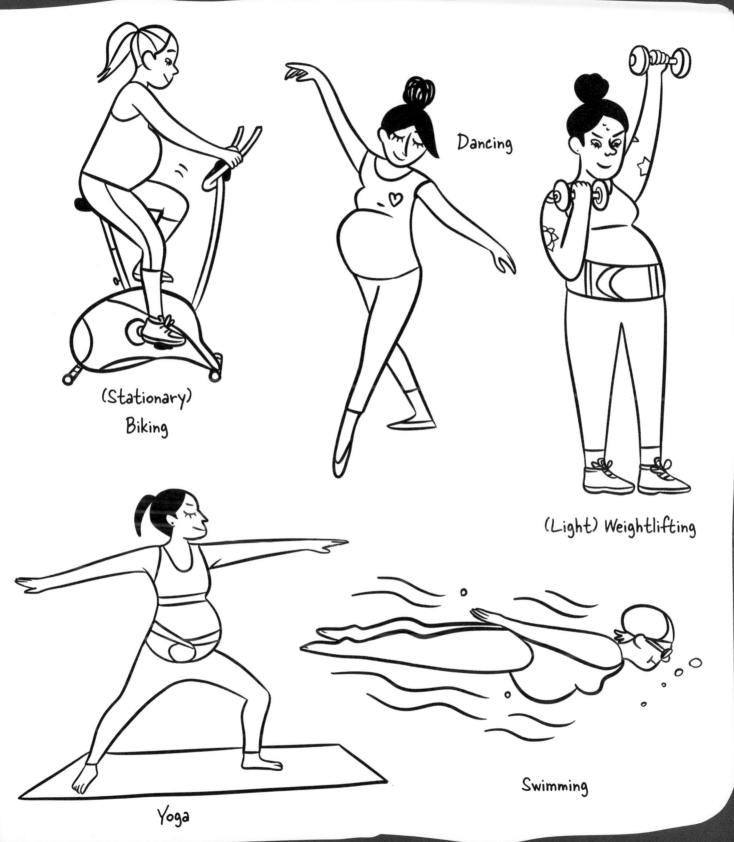

(Stationary)
Biking

Dancing

(Light) Weightlifting

Yoga

Swimming

WAYS YOU CAN (AND SHOULD) PAMPER YOURSELF RIGHT NOW

Think of it as self-care for two.

BELLY OIL	HANG WITH FRIENDS
MASSAGE	MEDITATE
FACIAL	EAT
BATH	SHOP
FUZZY SLIPPERS	GO TO THE MOVIES
COMFY ROBE	TAKE A TRIP
MANICURE	JOURNAL
PEDICURE	SIT
HAIRCUT	NAP
READ	NAP AGAIN

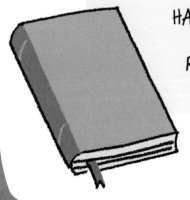

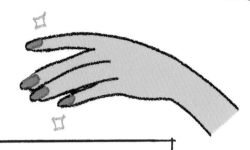

```
T W B T F F X P C Q V G W N I K G C O
J H M R R U A M A N I C U R E O O Z H
I G E E N Z Y A Y B A N Q A A T A V
M C O V B W R Z O S V Y D F U L O S Z
P F D X R U O H Y G S E F O Q V T R P
E B A T H B A A M S V A L L Y Y Y H P
D M A F G E H N W I L T G K G M E A L
I X F K R L S G W D G I E P E R M P K
C V N F T L Q W I J N D P C Y A O A F
U U N I D Y E I H O W G J P V T V G Q
R Q J E L O B T R R E A D Y E W I A W
E V A R X I L H O Z H Y N N W R E I N
B P H D X L L F A D X U X Q L J S N D
T Y C O M F Y R O B E A Z U G E S C I
J B B Y D Q H I T A K E A T R I P I O
K H S V Y K L E I P T E Q K R S E E T
H A I R C U T N P M J O X K V J P L K
S H O P J M E D I T A T E F A C I A L
R B M N L D B S H J O U R N A L B C R
```

Answers on page 94.

NURSERY THEMES

Honestly, we didn't know baby nursery themes were a thing until we got lost in Pinterest for several hours (days? What month is it?). But if you don't have years to spend looking at wall hangings, just take the following quiz and then see page 94 to find out what the theme of your baby's nursery should be!

1. **Where do you look for design inspo?**
   a. The zoo
   b. The night sky
   c. The mountains
   d. Transylvania

2. **The palette you're envisioning is:**
   a. Colorful
   b. Dark
   c. Earth tones
   d. Pitch black

3. **What kind of curtains are we thinking?**
   a. Animal print
   b. Stars
   c. Something that reminds me of a forest canopy
   d. Basically capes

4. **How about wall hangings?**
   a. Animal decals
   b. Moons
   c. A mural of mountains
   d. A bunch of sconces

5. **If you could choose one ridiculously oversized plush, what would it be?**
   a. A giraffe
   b. A rocket ship
   c. A grizzly bear
   d. A vampire bat

6. **If you hang a cross-stitch on the wall, it'll say:**
   a. "Let's get wild!"
   b. "To infinity and beyond"
   c. "The great outdoors"
   d. "I want to suck your blood"

Answers on page 94.

7. **If you imagine a song playing in the nursery, it's:**
   a. Anything from *The Lion King*
   b. Anything from *Star Wars*
   c. Ambient water sounds
   d. Foreboding organ music

8. **Who is your style icon?**
   a. Anyone wearing leopard print
   b. Sally Ride
   c. Reese Witherspoon in the movie *Wild*
   d. Count Dracula

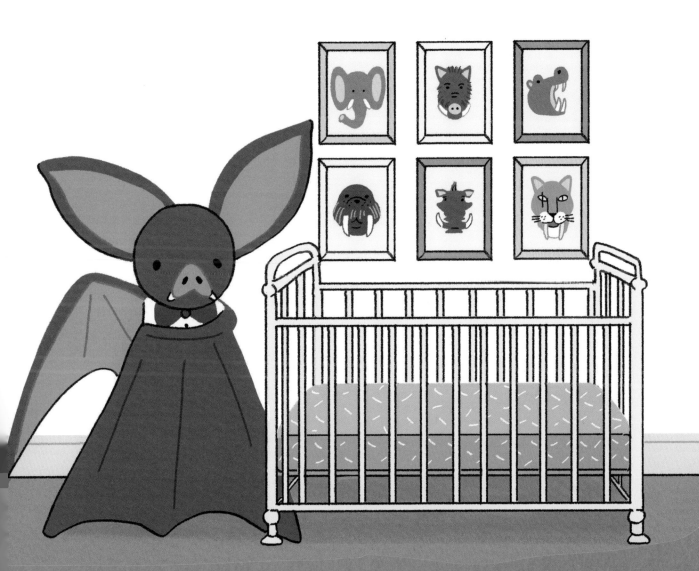

TRAVELING WHILE PREGNANT

Whether you're planning a babymoon or traveling for your partner's friend's wedding, here are some tips to help keep you comfortable-ish.

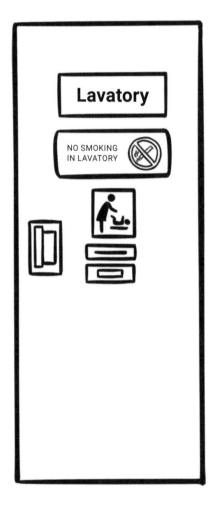

Get an aisle seat, for ease of peeing.

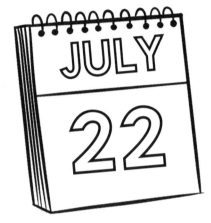

If you're flying, check the calendar to make sure you still can.

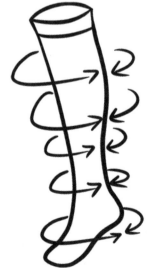

Wear compression socks, for blood flow.

Bring nausea remedies . . .

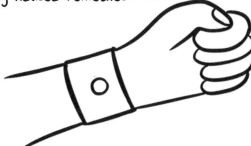

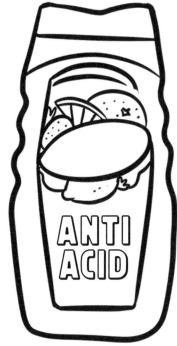

. . . and also gas remedies.

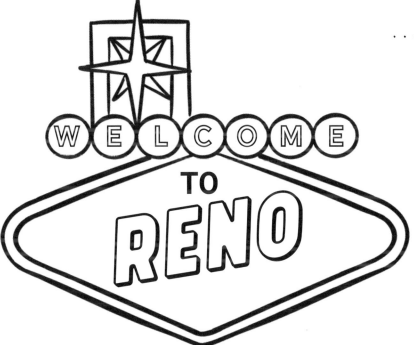

Find out where the local hospital is, in case your baby decides they want to be born in Reno.

GREETINGS FROM BABYMOON

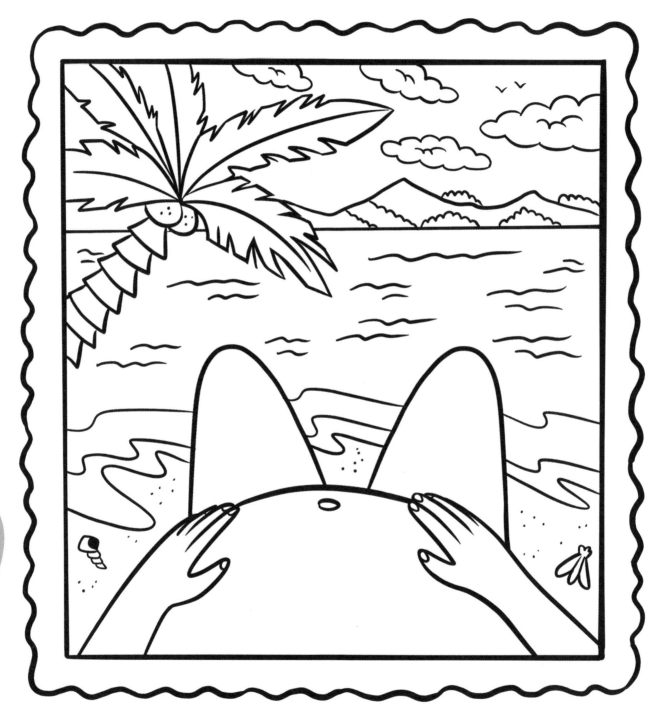

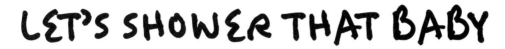

LET'S SHOWER THAT BABY

If you've got a chill friend or relative whom you trust to plan your baby shower, that's great. But if you think your loved one might need a little help, fill out this page, silently hand it to them, and walk away.

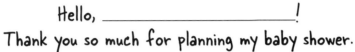

Hello, _____!
Thank you so much for planning my baby shower.

My favorite snacks are _____.

My favorite desserts are _____.

Foods that currently make me feel nauseous/gassy/grossed out are

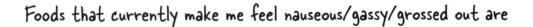

_____.

I would like to play baby shower games. Yes / No
(Circle one)

Make sure you invite _____.

Make sure you do <u>not</u> invite _____.

The time of day I like to take naps right now is

_____.

Thanks again! You are a great
Relative / Friend / Person I Just Met on the Street.
(Circle one)

SHOWER CRASHERS

We hope this isn't how your shower goes, but if it does, it'll make a great story! If you've got a buddy nearby, hand this page to them so they can write your answers in. Or if you're flying solo, do your best to fill them in without peeking at the story first. You heard us, no peeking!

You'll never believe what happened at my baby shower this weekend. I was thanking my

friend _____ for the _____ they gifted
        (NAME OF YOUR BEST FRIEND)   (BABY ITEM)

me, when out of nowhere, _____ walks in. I was completely
                              (CELEBRITY NAME)

_____! Not only did they basically become best friends with my
        (EMOTION)

_____, but they ate all of the _____
        (RELATIVE)   (TYPE OF PASTRY, PLURAL)

my coworker baked! They drank all of the _____ too!
                                              (COCKTAIL OR MOCKTAIL, PLURAL)

But they were so _____, I just couldn't be mad at them.
                        (EMOTION)

In fact, I told them I'd name my baby after them. So that's how

I ended up naming my child _____ Jr.!
                                  (SAME CELEBRITY)

BABY SHOWER DESSERTS

Just wanted to take another moment to think about desserts and color them in.

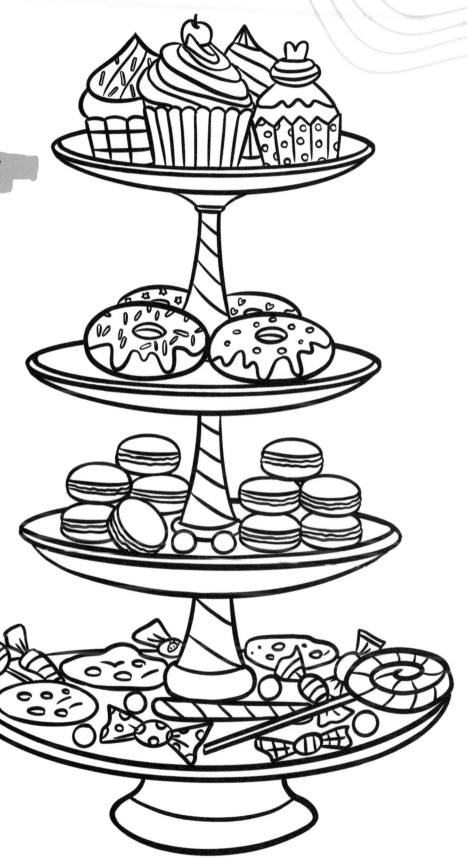

MATERNITY WARDROBE STAPLES

Figuring out what to wear while your body is changing so rapidly can be daunting. But have no fear, leggings are here. Color in your new wardrobe!

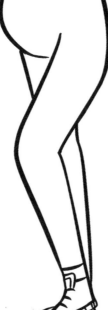

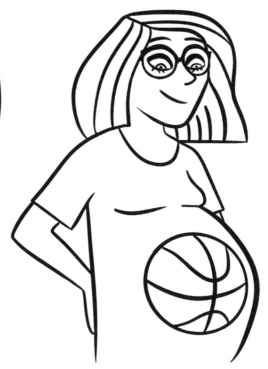

High-waisted leggings. And make 'em stretchy.

Big T-shirts. For day, night, and everything in between.

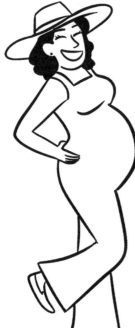

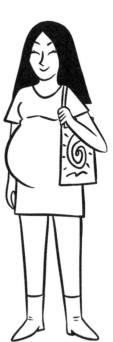

Jumpsuits. Upside: you don't have to pick out a shirt and pants. Downside: really hard to pee.

Shirtdresses. Like a jumpsuit, but easier for peeing.

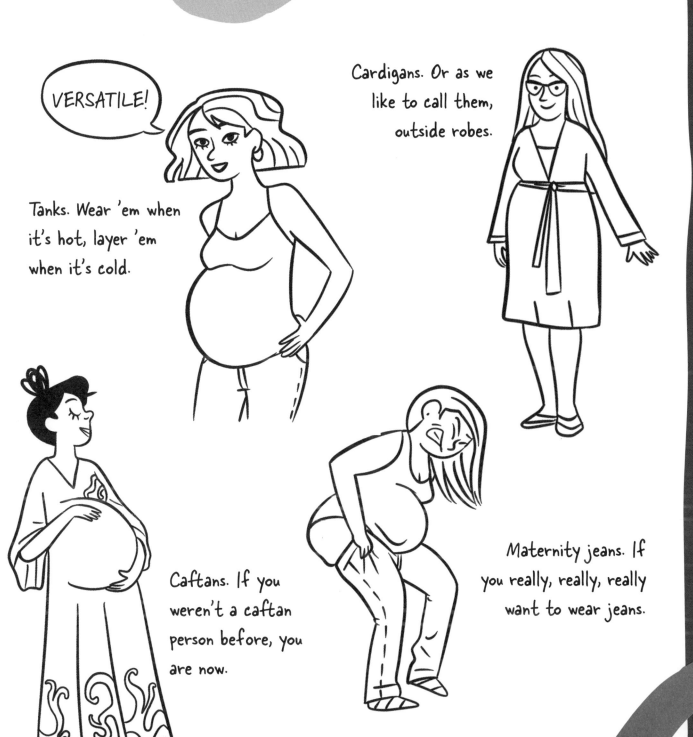

VERSATILE!

Tanks. Wear 'em when it's hot, layer 'em when it's cold.

Cardigans. Or as we like to call them, outside robes.

Caftans. If you weren't a caftan person before, you are now.

Maternity jeans. If you really, really, really want to wear jeans.

ALL THE NURSERY STUFF

Wow, there's a lot of baby stuff! Sure, your baby might not really need everything listed here, but if you want to get all this *and* a life-size teddy bear, we're not gonna stop you.

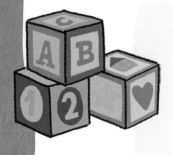

CRIB	BOOKS
CHANGING TABLE	SHEETS
ROCKING CHAIR	MATTRESS
SOUND MACHINE	BOUNCER
NIGHT-LIGHT	SWADDLE BLANKETS
DIAPER PAIL	DIAPERS
DRESSER	WIPES
BOOKSHELF	FEEDING PILLOW
BABY MONITOR	PLAY MAT
TOYS	DIAPER CREAM

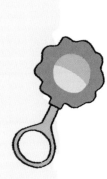

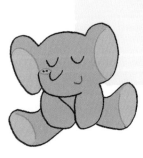

```
H E D X T X L L L Z B C L E T A M J W S C N E
W D I V U G B Z M E L W L H B K F A M E W S H
I I A T T G I I I J Q B R T E R B W W Z T J B
Q A P N H C F W O L A N Z R V I C C D I T I S
H P E U O A E U D T V N V I M U T H X I R B H
R E R Z O T E P G P R K B F D R D G M C X B S
E R P Q L E D N N F L I F K A Q Y A Z S Q O W
S C A M J Q I H I P C A B U N N W Q H M D O A
R R I R F G N X M G J M Y Y V E M Q Q D R K D
U E L V N U G A A Y H Z H M A G X O P O M S D
B A K A C V P M T C V T R B A A T L T H P H L
P M H X X C I Z T V S I L Y O T P I E S I E E
B C B L N J L J R S H A A I L T N L R B F L B
O I E I V P L B E J K L K V G O J E R T D F L
U X L L J N O X S D S Y G Y M H S Y H R N B A
N U G R R N W M S D D A D Y Z S T I R F T B N
C V Q G U N K G G M P E B T E O U H U S F O K
E T R O C K I N G C H A I R S T O Y S Y A O E
R L D G S J S Y V X B J D R G H U H B C F K T
D I A E D D I A P E R S O K Z B E T R W V S S
U Z P E Q Z P Z X A R W D I Z H M E K B Y U Q
W I V K L Q T H X Z I F W V D L T I T W X L L
W S O U N D M A C H I N E A I F I C I S U U H
```

Answers on page 95.

POINT A TO POINT B(ABY)

Okay, *very* no pressure, but at some point you're actually going to have this baby. Make sure to do a dry run of getting to the hospital or birthing center or wherever it's happening, as you never know what might pop up along the way!

START →

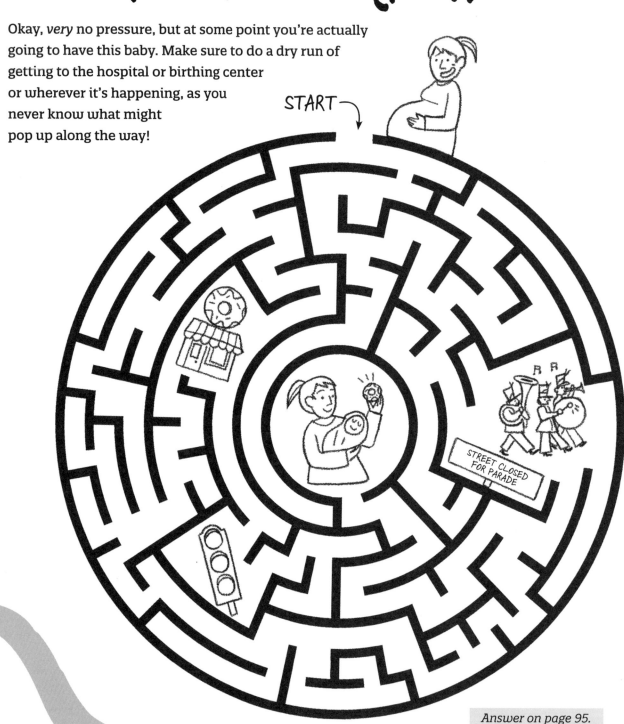

Answer on page 95.

SENSIBLE SANDALS

Color in your new shoes because your top priorities right now are comfort, shoes that fit, and not having to tie laces.

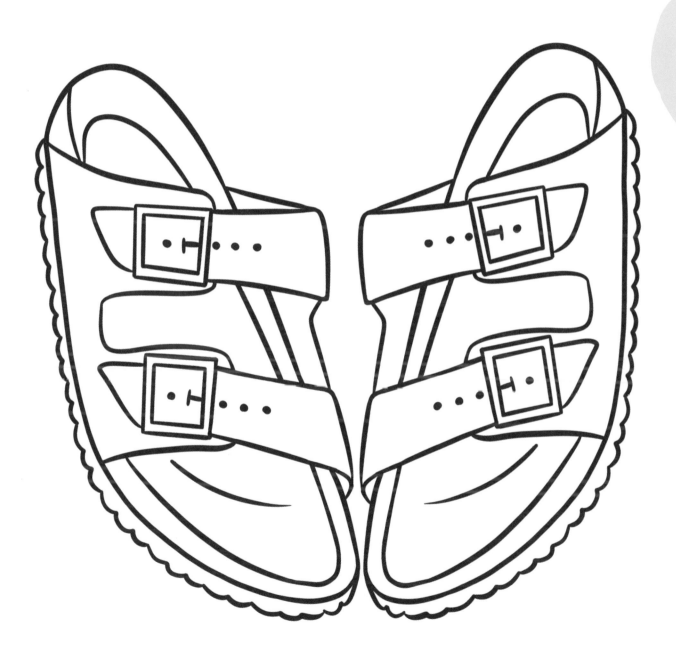

GET COMFY

See how many words you can create using the phrase "Stretchy pants are my friend."
For example, "fetch." Or "party." Okay, now it just sounds like we're at a birthday party
for a dog, and that's just delightful.

Stretchy pants are my friend.

_____   _____

_____   _____

_____   _____

_____   _____

_____   _____

_____   _____

_____   _____

_____   _____

_____   _____

ANATOMY OF A DIAPER BAG

Sooner rather than later, you will be mid–diaper change at a restaurant wondering where the wipes are. But until then, memorize everything you'll need to fit in your diaper bag, then flip the page and see if you can answer the questions about it.

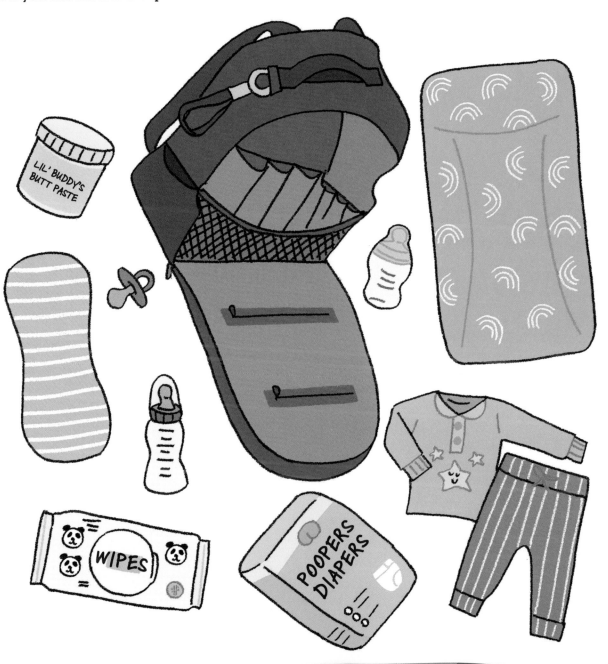

NOW TEST YOUR MEMORY

Think about the picture you studied on the previous page, and answer as many of these questions as you can!

What was the brand of diapers? _____

How many baby bottles were there? _____

What pattern was on the changing mat? _____

What brand was the diaper-rash cream? _____

What pattern was on the burp cloth? _____

How many items were there total? _____

What did you forget to pack? _____

Answers on page 95.

BYE BYE, SITTING

While we're sure you're thrilled to welcome your bundle of joy, we want to give you a very chill heads-up that once they're here, you might not have time for some of the things you usually enjoy. Unscramble this list of activities that we recommend you cherish while you're able.

AEGNVIL EHT UEHSO TA THING

_____ _____ _____ _____ _____

GINKTA A NOGL REWOHS _____ _____ _____

RINDKING ECFEOF HLIWE S'TI THO

_____ _____ _____ _____ _____

GBENI NLAOE _____ _____   SEIHBOB _____

NGIDO TIHNNOG _____ _____

ACNGIHTW VT _____ _____

YILNG NWDO _____ _____

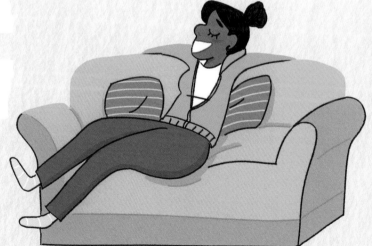

Answers on page 95.

WHAT'S IN A NAME?

Kind of a lot, it turns out! So here are some questions you can ask yourself to help guide you on your name-choosing journey.

Do you want a name that's gender-specific or gender-neutral?

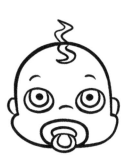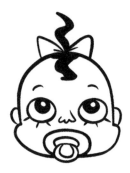

How about popular vs. unique?

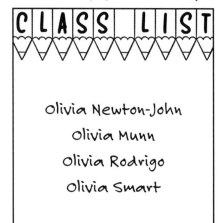

CLASS LIST

Olivia Newton-John

Olivia Munn

Olivia Rodrigo

Olivia Smart

Are there any family names you might want to use (including your own, Gilmore Girls style)?

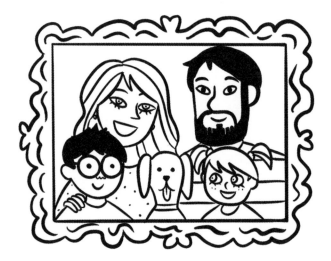

How about artists you admire?

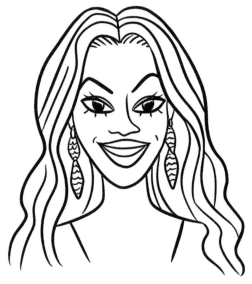

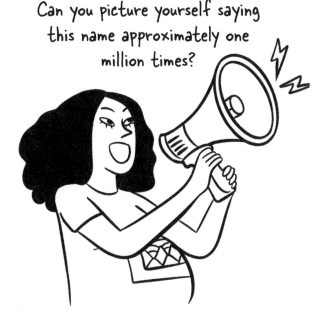

Can you picture yourself saying this name approximately one million times?

Who are your enemies? (Also, okay, wow, there are a lot of them!)

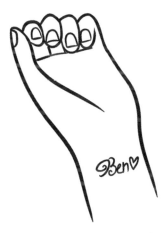

Would you get a necklace or tattoo of it?

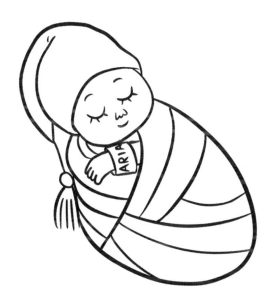

When your baby is born, can you look at them and say, "They're such a(n) _____." (I guess this is a question for future you!)

DRESS FOR THE OCCASION

Dressing for special occasions isn't that different when you're pregnant, except that none of your clothes fit and you're carrying a human in your body. Feel free to actually cut out the paper doll and outfits or just color for funsies!

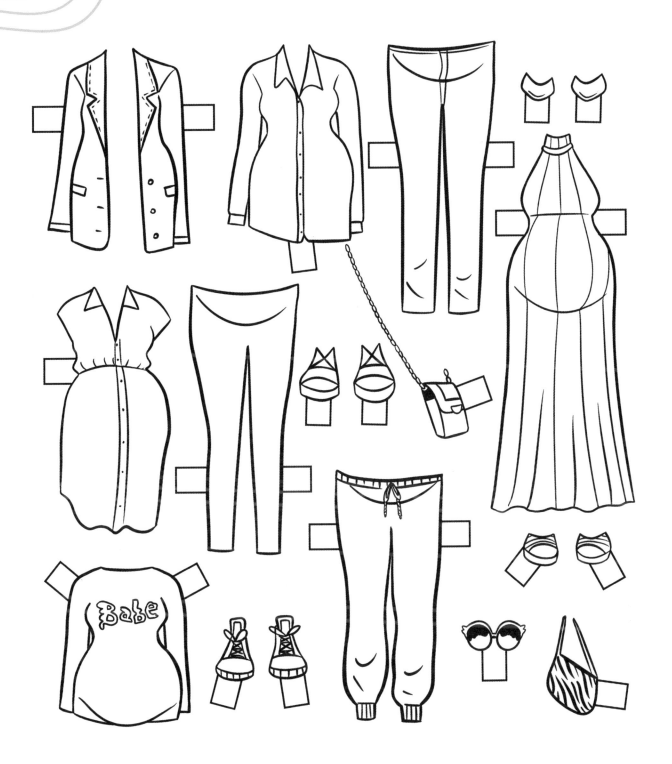

BIRTH PLANNING

Okay, wow, turns out there are a lot of decisions to make when it comes to delivering a baby! Only you know what's right for you, but here are some things that may (or may not!) be on your birth plan.

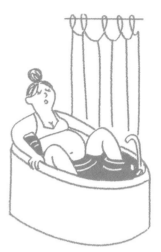

VAGINAL

C-SECTION

HOSPITAL

HOME BIRTH

BIRTHING CENTER

MOVE AROUND

DRINK FLUIDS

BIRTH BALL

SHOWER

BATH

BREASTFEED

BOTTLE FEED

MIRROR

PLACENTA

EPIDURAL

LIGHTS DIMMED

EYE DROPS

INDUCTION

PHOTOGRAPHY

SUPPORT PERSON

MONITORING

UMBILICAL CORD

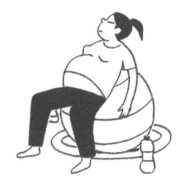

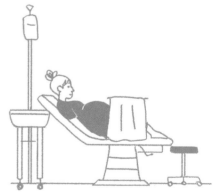

```
Q J A Y C L C J B U B C B Y L W S H O W E R S
E S N O U Q C C H I N Q U I L O H O I M M W N
S D Y D R Q D G P H R D X M N R M S Y J Q X O
J W X M J R B I E Y X T C W E L I P K M Z H V
P H O T O G R A P H Y D H S D O T I W U E Z A
E D T B O T T L E F E E D I E F P T Z P B H G
P P R D E X W G Q B F T F T N C P A R L T A I
C M I I S L O Y W R G K W M X G T L W A O F N
Y I N D N I J K Q Y E B T N P H C I B C D Z A
W H H S U K J O T R Q L O S T U D E O E Q I L
P Q Y U B R F Z Y D O I S R E N G M N N K Q A
F U J P H K A L G Y T E I E U X O C D T K Y L
M B H P F S O L U C T B W O R J N E D A E L T
O R X O A N O D U I E R R D Z M M M R B A R E
N E P R Q B M D A M D A C B P M Z T M B P R Y
I A Q T R Q N I O Y E S H R I F E S H F P V E
T S D P Q I K H R V X L R D N F R T S V X G D
O T W E L U T E O R N N S F J Q R D G G F W R
R F X R F D J M W E O T V O V I O Q L Y R W O
I E D S H J S T E Z H R D Q B W M B G C F G P
N E U O F R P A N G L L H C Y K N O Y D L H S
G D W N V U M B I L I C A L C O R D K G H A V
Q F J S A T Q L I F E K B S P K R S B O Y H T
```

Answers on page 95.

DANCE PARTY!

When you have a baby, the meaning of the phrase "dance party" can change drastically. Spot the differences between how your current nights out and future nights in might look, and color them in!

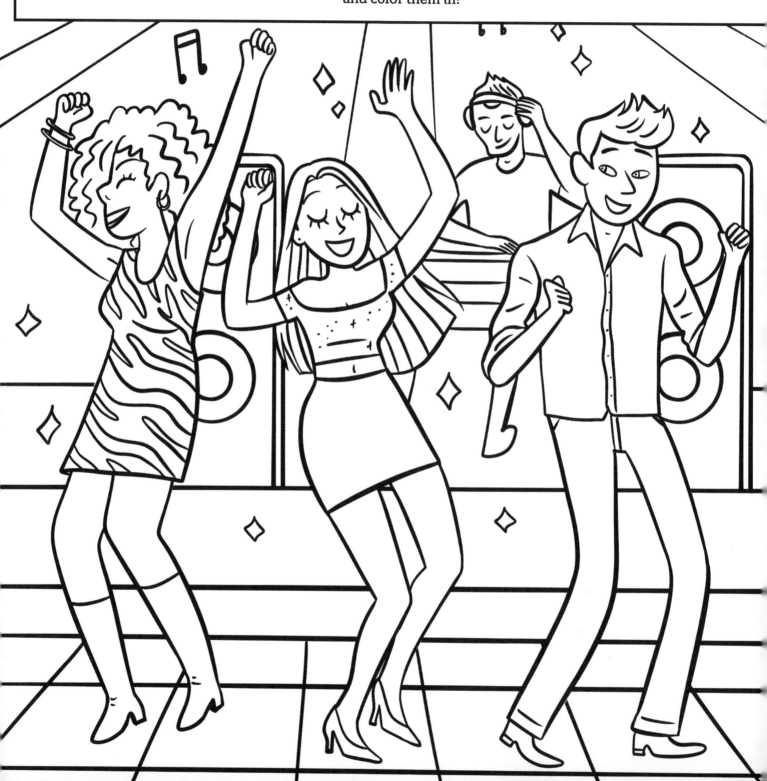

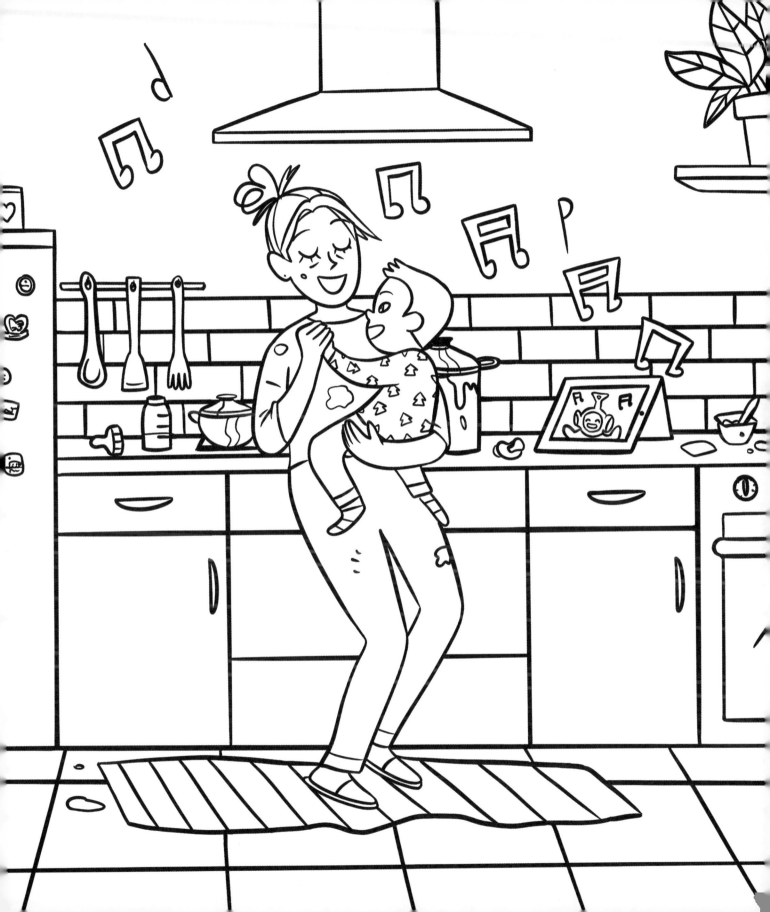

SPICE UP YOUR SWADDLE

You're gonna have to do a lot of swaddling once baby is here, and using the same technique over and over again can get boring. So why not mix it up a little and try a few of these? On second thought, maybe just color them in.

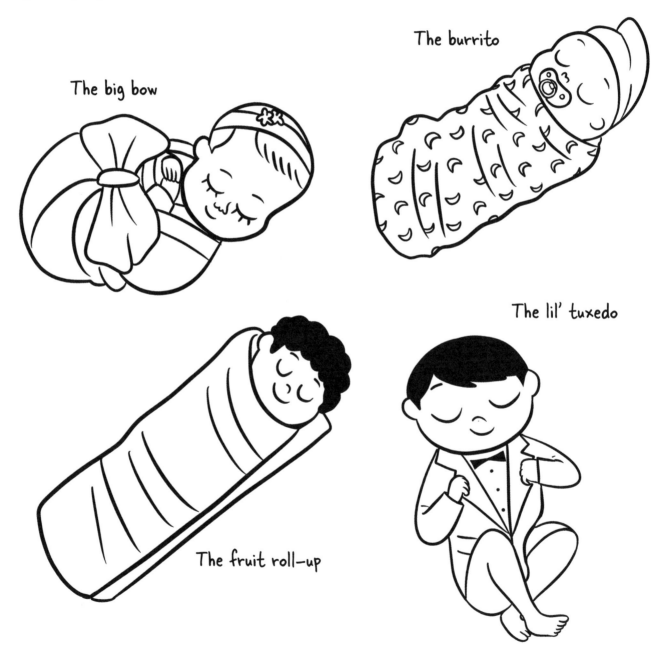

The burrito

The big bow

The lil' tuxedo

The fruit roll-up

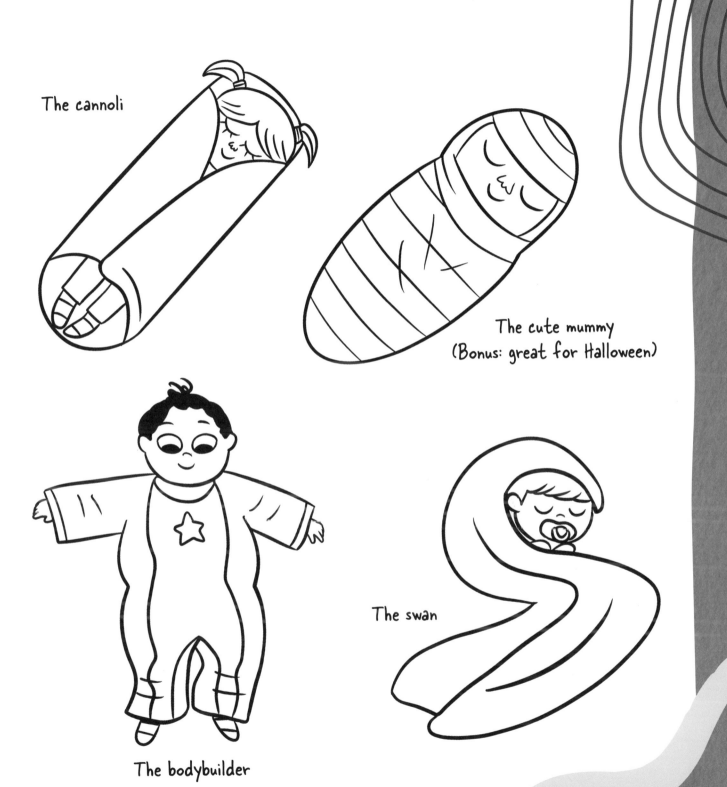

The cannoli

The cute mummy
(Bonus: great for Halloween)

The bodybuilder

The swan

USEFUL MANTRAS FOR CHILDBIRTH

Thinking about actually getting the baby out of there can be a little scary, so here are some helpful mantras you can use before or during your birth.

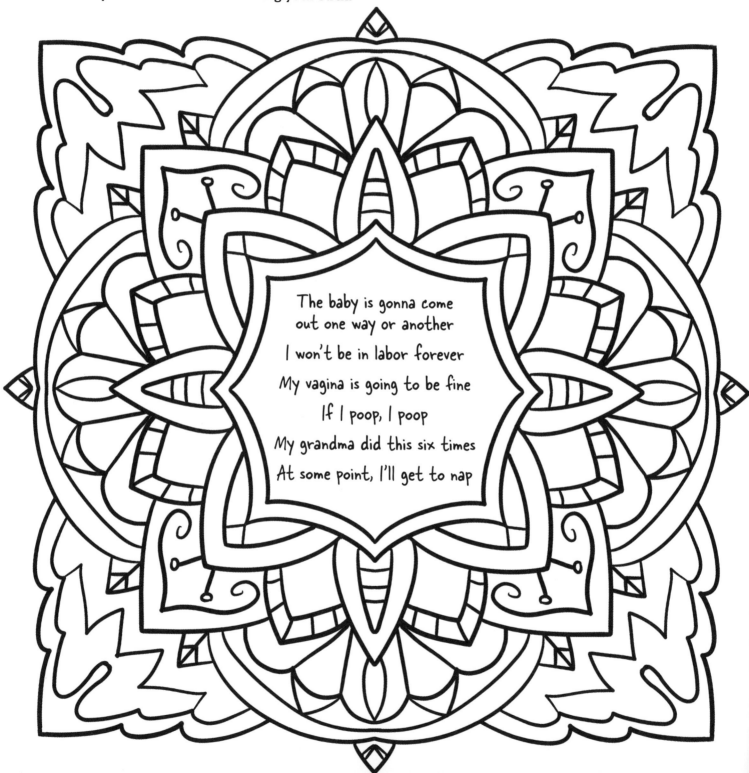

The baby is gonna come out one way or another

I won't be in labor forever

My vagina is going to be fine

If I poop, I poop

My grandma did this six times

At some point, I'll get to nap

HAHA, OKAY, BUT SERIOUSLY, GET THIS BABY OUT OF HERE

As you get closer to your due date (or past it), it's understandable to feel very over being pregnant. So unscramble the following methods of inducing labor naturally, which aren't guaranteed to work but are maybe worth a try?

SICXEERE _____

NGEATI SETDA
_____

XSE _____

REUSACPSURE
_____

REUTCACPUUN
_____

PPLNIE ULNOITASTIM
_____

GAESSAM
_____

NIAETG YCIPS OOSFD
_____

Answers on page 95.

YOU'RE GOING HOME, BABY!

Pretend that a non-creepy, well-meaning stranger has a Polaroid camera when you're leaving the hospital, and show us your and baby's going-home outfits!

ANSWER KEY

Get That Salad Away from Me!
page 9

EGGS

ONIONS

FISH

GARLIC

MEAT

SPICY FOODS

DAIRY PRODUCTS

COFFEE

It's 12 a.m., Do You Know Where Your Curly Fries Are?
page 10

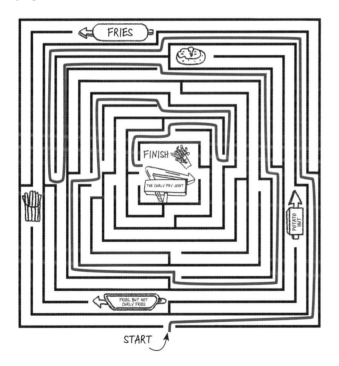

True or False: What's Off-Limits
page 12

1. False. Caffeine is fine in moderation. And by moderation, we mean up to two cups of coffee. Some evidence even shows that up to four cups is okay.

2. False. One or two drinks a week in the first trimester and up to one drink a day in the second and third trimesters seems to be a-okay, but binge drinking should definitely be avoided.

3. False. The types of bacteria that could be present when eating raw fish aren't any more dangerous when you're pregnant than when you're not. Maybe exercise caution, but sushi isn't off-limits completely.

4. True. Smoking, even moderately, can negatively affect your baby.

5. Also true, although more research is needed about marijuana in pregnancy.

6. True, sort of. It depends on the cheese. If the cheese is pasteurized, it's okay to eat. Just check the label, or if you're at a restaurant, make sure to ask.

7. False. Rare meats are off-limits due to risk of contracting toxoplasmosis. And actually, the same infection can be caused by unwashed fruits and vegetables, so make sure you wash yours well!

8. False, mostly. The concern with deli meats is listeria exposure. Listeria does grow well at refrigerator temperature, but the biggest culprit, deli-meats-wise, has been deli turkey. Good to exercise caution here as well, though!

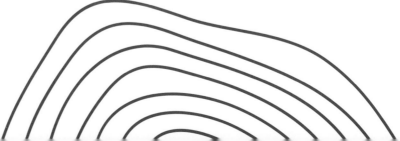

All the Feels
page 18

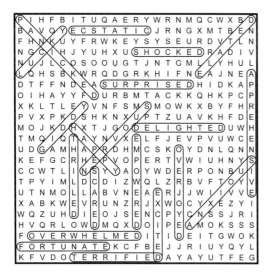

Find Your Phone
page 21

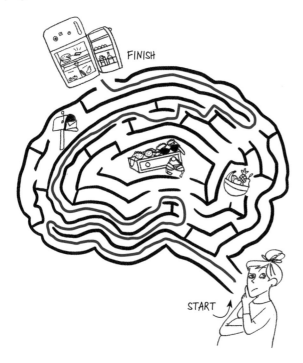

Actually, Really Great Things about Being Pregnant
page 24

NO PERIOD

GREAT HAIR

STRONG NAILS

STRANGERS ARE NICE

BABY KICKS

ELASTIC WAISTBANDS

FEELING EMPOWERED

SO MANY NAPS

Wait, I Can't Go Skydiving?
page 30

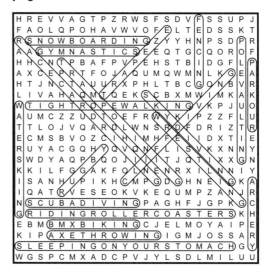

Where Should You 'Moon?
page 32

If you answered mostly As, then get on a plane and head to a great hiking destination! A national park, a mountain, a canyon. We don't know how you still have so much energy, but hey, that's great!

If you answered mostly Bs, head to a big city. Take in the sights, try to ignore the smells, and enjoy being at a museum pre-having a small child.

If you answered mostly Cs, hit the beach! Put up your feet, get a massage, and make good use of that on-premises restaurant.

If you answered mostly Ds, try a staycation. Book a hotel nearby, order room service, enjoy those sweet, sweet hotel pillows, and watch as much TV as you want. Not that you need us to tell you that you can watch lots of TV, but like, watch lots of TV.

Things That Make You Pee Now, Apparently
page 36

SNEEZING	COUGHING
LAUGHING	BENDING
RUNNING	LIFTING
WALKING	EVERYTHING

So What Are They Doing in There?
page 40

1. True. They may even be able to hear your heartbeat as early as 18 weeks. Do they just think you're constantly playing the drums? There's no way to know for sure.

2. True. This happens later in pregnancy, and they're mostly just seeing light, but hey, pretty cool!

3. True. They'll be able to taste what you're eating via their amniotic fluid, especially if it's a strong flavor.

4. False. As far as we know, babies do not know what chicken tikka masala is in the womb.

5. True. And they sleep a lot. Like, they are sleeping most of the time. Must be nice, huh?

6. True. Well, babies in the womb experience REM sleep, which is usually when dreaming happens. But fun to think about a lil' baby dreaming about, I dunno, puppies??

7. True. Smell is one of the first senses to develop.

8. False. Sorry, babies.

Here's Your Kicker
page 44

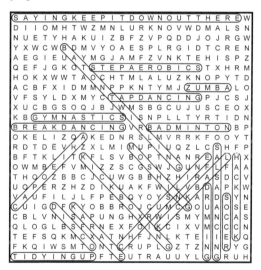

Wait, New Undies Too??
page 48

If you answered mostly As, your maternity underwear vibe is Sporty! You're cool and confident and would probably know what to do if a stray volleyball were headed in your direction. You're still pretty active (good for you!), and you want to keep your growing body supported as you move around.

If you answered mostly Bs, your vibe is Comfy! You're very go-with-the-flow and only check your email a few times a day. You're a relaxed parent-to-be and your underwear reflects that.

If you answered mostly Cs, your vibe is Sexy! You're in the bedroom regularly, and not just for sleep. You've got it, you flaunt it, and you even know what "it" is.

If you answered mostly Ds, your vibe is Granny! You never leave the house after 8 p.m. and sometimes you're even in bed by then. You take comfort to the next level, and honestly? We're here for it.

The Moods, They Are A-Changin'
page 51

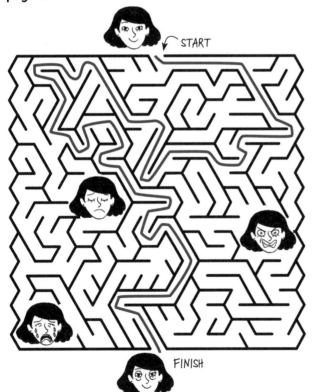

Ways You Can (and Should) Pamper Yourself Right Now
page 58

```
T W B T F F X P C Q V G W N I K G C O
J H M R R U A M A N I C U R E O O Z H
I G E E E N Z Y A Y B A N Q A A T A V
M C O V B W R Z O S V Y D F U L O S Z
P F D X R U O H Y G S E F O Q V T R P
E B A T H B A A M S V A L L Y Y H N P
D M A F G E H N W I L T G K G M E A L
I X F K R L S G W D G I P E P R M P K
C V N F T L Q W I J N D P C Y A O A F
U U N I D Y E I H O W G J P V T V G Q
R Q J E L O B T R R E A D Y E W I I A W
E V A R X I L H O Z H Y N N W R E I N
B P H D X U L F A D X U X Q L J S N D
T Y C O M F Y R O B E A Z U G E S C I
J B B Y D Q H I T A K E A T R I P I O
K H S V Y K L E I P T E Q K R S E E T
H A I R C U T N P M J O X K V J P L K
S H O P J M E D I T A T E F A C I A L
R B M N L D B S H J O U R N A L B C R
```

Nursery Themes
page 60

If you answered mostly As, then your nursery theme is Animals! You want to bring the zoo to you.

If you answered mostly Bs, then your theme is Outer Space! You want a combination nursery/planetarium.

If your answered mostly Cs, your theme is Outdoorsy! Who needs to hike when the mountains are in your baby's room?

If you answered mostly Ds, your theme is Dracula! Are you an actual vampire? Possibly! Or maybe you're just into goth stuff. Regardless, it doesn't seem like anyone's ever done this theme for a baby nursery before, so you'd be the first and we love that for you.

All the Nursery Stuff
page 70

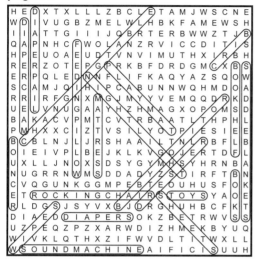

Point A to Point B(aby)
page 72

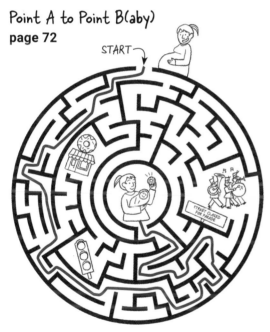

Anatomy of a Diaper Bag
page 76

POOPERS

TWO

RAINBOWS

LIL' BUDDY'S BUTT PASTE

STRIPES

ELEVEN

YOUR PHONE, BUT WHERE IS IT ANYWAY? SEE PAGE 21.

Bye, Bye Sitting
page 77

LEAVING THE HOUSE AT NIGHT

TAKING A LONG SHOWER

DRINKING COFFEE WHILE IT'S HOT

BEING ALONE

HOBBIES

DOING NOTHING

WATCHING TV

LYING DOWN

Birth Planning
page 82

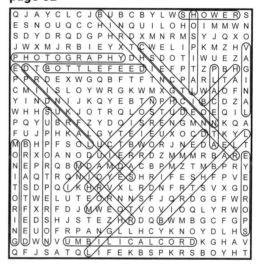

Haha, Okay, But Seriously, Get This Baby Out of Here
page 89

EXERCISE

EATING DATES

SEX

ACUPRESSURE

ACUPUNCTURE

NIPPLE STIMULATION

MASSAGE

EATING SPICY FOODS

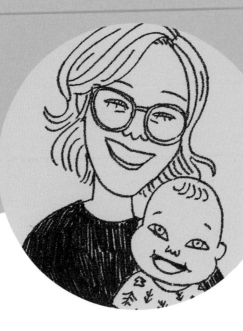

ABOUT THE AUTHOR

RACHEL HASTINGS is a writer in the Los Angeles area. She is originally from Wilkes-Barre, Pennsylvania, and studied Television-Radio at Ithaca College in upstate New York. She then moved to the west coast, where she wrote sketch comedy at the Upright Citizens Brigade Theater. She primarily works in television, and her credits include *Bob's Burgers* (FOX), *The Fungies* (Cartoon Network), *Central Park* (Apple TV+), and *Praise Petey* (Freeform). She also contributed to the *Bob's Burgers* Comic Book. She lives in Burbank with her husband and one-year-old son, both of whom greatly inspired the content of this book.